Nursing Peer Review

A Practical, Nonpunitive Approach to Case Review

Laura Cook Harrington, RN, BSN, MHA, CPHQ, CPCQM
Marla Smith, MHSA

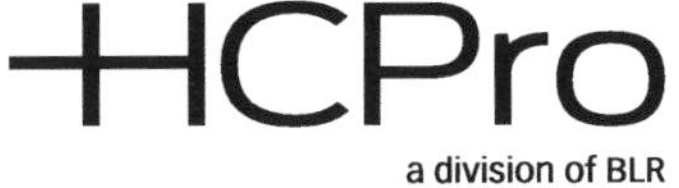

a division of BLR

Nursing Peer Review, Second Edition is published by HCPro, a division of BLR

 5 4 3 2 1

Download the additional materials of this book at *www.hcpro.com/downloads/12285*

ISBN: 978-1-55645-198-0

HCPro provides information resources for the healthcare industry.

Laura Cook Harrington, RN, BSN, MHA, CPHQ, CPCQM, Author
Marla Smith, MHSA, Author
Claudette Moore, Acquisitions Editor
Rebecca Hendren, Product Manager
Erin Callahan, Senior Director, Product
Elizabeth Petersen, Vice President
Matt Sharpe, Production Supervisor
Vincent Skyers, Design Manager
Vicki McMahan, Sr. Graphic Designer/Layout
Jason Gregory, Cover Designer

Arrangements can be made for quantity discounts. For more information, contact:
HCPro
75 Sylvan Street, Suite A-101
Danvers, MA 01923
Telephone: 800-650-6787 or 781-639-1872
Fax: 800-639-8511
Email: *customerservice@hcpro.com*

Visit HCPro online at: *www.hcpro.com* and *www.hcmarketplace.com*

Contents

List of Figures

Nursing Continuing Education

For information on earning **3.5** hours of Continuing Nursing Education credits, and to download additional materials supporting this book, visit your downloads page: *www.hcpro.com/downloads/12285*.

Learning objectives for *Nursing Peer Review, Second Edition:*

1. Identify three external sources imposing higher standards for reporting nursing quality performance
2. Discuss the traditional structure for reviewing complaints about nurses
3. Describe three different categories of performance review
4. Explain the differences between peer oversight and peer review
5. List four goals of conducting peer review
6. Identify elements included in the dimensions of performance
7. Describe the performance pyramid model
8. Describe the three types of peer review protection laws
9. Describe the components of the Health Care Quality and Improvement Act of 1986
10. Name two ways of protecting peer review information
11. List the advantages for creating a formalized structure to support peer review
12. Identify three goals of the nursing peer review committee
13. Describe the case review process relating to committee review
14. Identify referral sources for case reviews
15. List the process steps to take when care is deemed "appropriate" and "inappropriate"
16. Relate the importance of educating nurses and nonnurse stakeholders on the peer review process
17. Identify communication methods that are effective during the implementation process
18. List ways to reduce fear among nurses regarding the peer review process
19. List the different components of the case review form
20. Identify when a case would need further review by a clinical expert
21. Describe why it is important to track and trend data on a continual basis
22. List the different types of indicators used to evaluate nursing performance

23. Determine where indicator data is housed and how to extract it
24. Identify different types of feedback reports
25. Identify the next steps to improve performance when there are outliers based on data outcomes
26. Describe internal forces driving case review
27. Explain how a professional peer review process supports the "14 Forces of Magnetism," as identified by the American Nurses Credentialing Center (ANCC)

About the Authors

Laura Cook Harrington, RN, BSN, MHA, CPHQ, CHCQM

Laura Cook Harrington, RN, BSN, MHA, CPHQ, CHCQM, is the executive director of quality and patient safety at Boston Medical Center. Previously, she was the director of live events and continuing education and senior consultant at The Greeley Company, a division of HCPro. She is an experienced healthcare manager with extensive background in the areas of performance improvement, peer review, risk, case management, and credentialing.

Harrington is a registered nurse, a certified professional in healthcare quality, and a fellow of the American Board of Quality Assurance & Utilization Review Physicians. Harrington graduated from Texas Woman's University with a bachelor's degree in nursing and a master's degree in healthcare administration.

Marla Smith, MHSA

Marla Smith, MHSA, serves as a consultant for HCPro. Her areas of expertise are in medical staff and nursing peer review, medical and hospital quality performance improvement, and physician- and hospital-based data analysis. Prior to working with HCPro, Smith worked closely with clients during the assessment and restructuring of medical staff and hospital quality programs for The Greeley Company. Currently, she works with clients in the development and implementation of HCPro's Peer Review Case Tracking and Physician Profile Reporter databases.

About the Authors

Prior to working with HCPro and The Greeley Company, Smith worked for several years with a healthcare system in the Denver area in its health information management department and the medical staff office. Smith graduated from Regis University in Denver with an undergraduate degree in health information management and a graduate degree in health services administration.

Introduction

The term "peer review" is cropping up everywhere in today's healthcare environment, particularly when talk turns to quality care and standards of practice. It seems odd that much of nursing has yet to catch up to our medical staff brethren in terms of evaluating individual standards and quality of care, which is something medical staffs have been practicing for decades.

Peer review is about nurses taking responsibility for their practice and about nurses evaluating nurses. It is about raising the standards of practice for all, and ultimately about providing the best care we can for our patients.

If the profession of nursing does not focus on nurse performance—if nursing peer review programs are nonexistent or ineffective—then we run the risk of other entities taking control of the process for us. The best solution to this problem is to create or strengthen the nursing peer review process.

The goals and benefits of peer review include:

- Improving the quality of care provided by individual nurses
- Monitoring the performance of nurses
- Identifying opportunities for performance improvement
- Identifying systemwide issues
- Identifying educational needs of nurses

This book will walk you through everything you need to know to structure your own program and launch it with success. The chapters cover a five-step process:

1. Designing a committee
2. Establishing the process
3. Educating your organization
4. Implementing the program and conducting chart review
5. Tracking and trending data to establish benchmarks

Evaluating individual nurse performance should become an expectation for nursing as we strive to always improve the standard of nursing care we provide our patients.

Chapter 1

Defining Incident-Based Peer Review

Learning objectives

After reading this chapter, the participant will be able to:

- Identify three external sources imposing higher standards for reporting nursing quality performance
- Discuss the traditional structure for reviewing complaints about nurses
- Describe three different types of performance review
- Explain the differences between peer oversight and peer review
- Describe internal and external forces driving peer review

Peer review is a frequently used term in nursing, yet its connotations are many and varied. At its core, however, peer review relates to quality and improving standards of patient care through case review.

The Rise of Peer Review

As the nursing profession embraces efforts to improve practice, it must also align with the concept of evaluating individual standards and quality-of-care issues. Peer review allows such an evaluation in a safe, nonpunitive environment. It allows nurses to take control of their practice and to decide with their peers the quality standards to which they will hold themselves.

According to the American Nurses Association's *Nursing: Scope and Standards of Practice*, peer review is "a collegial, systematic, and periodic process by which RNs are held accountable for practice and which fosters the refinement of one's knowledge, skills, and decision-making at all levels and in all areas of practice" (2004).

While peer review is a growing practice in nursing, the methods for evaluating nurse quality of care and how quality-of-care issues are treated at different facilities is lacking. As a profession, we do want nurses to act in professional and competent manners, but we lack a formal structure with which to evaluate ongoing nurse performance.

The ANCC Magnet® Recognition Program: A focus on standards

As a process devoted to improving nurse performance and encouraging nurses to be accountable for their practice, peer review is a natural fit for many organizations pursuing American Nurses Credentialing Center (ANCC) Magnet Recognition Program® (MRP) designation, which recognizes facilities that have achieved a high standard of nursing excellence.

MRP emphasizes the need for "formal, informal, regular and ongoing performance appraisal processes," which naturally would include peer review It identifies how the peer review process may be used for "professional growth for nurses at all levels in the organization" and emphasizes "the value of establishing, monitoring, and evaluating practice standards."

GO TO › Chapter 11 discusses specific ways in which the MRP Forces of Magnet ism apply to nursing peer review.

Other external sources may impose high standards

Patient safety is an ongoing issue in healthcare, and consumers are increasingly aware of quality-of-care issues. In addition to the ANCC's MRP, other external sources such as The Joint Commission, healthcare insurance providers, patients, and payers increasingly expect higher-quality care and transparency in reporting. Although many of these demands are placed solely on doctors, it is only a matter of time before nurses are held to the same high level of accountability.

In fact, the emphasis on accountability in nursing has increased steadily for the past 25 years, and each day that a medical error is committed, the calls for nursing accountability grow louder. The trend toward public reporting of medical errors and healthcare data and the drive to increase transparency in healthcare are simply pushing accountability to the forefront. The nursing profession as a whole must take the reins and hold itself accountable.

Nursing leaders and decision-makers must spearhead the drive to create formal standards for evaluating ongoing nurse performance. These standards must be nonpunitive and impartial, so lessons may truly be learned about the educational needs of the nurses.

If we do not learn to evaluate ourselves, we risk being evaluated by others. By taking the lead, we can decide for ourselves the essential nursing values and standards rather than having them imposed on us by other, external forces.

How Facilities Use Peer Review

Organizations wanting to establish a program for evaluating nursing practice and raising standards must emphasize a nonpunitive culture. Without a *blameless culture*, organizations will experience selective incident reporting and hostility and resentment from nursing staff. Nonpunitive peer review offers a safe environment where nursing practice issues can be evaluated by nurses, where issues are discussed by those who understand what the nursing world is like, and where recommendations can be made that will be accepted and understood by the nursing staff.

Before creating a program, organizations must first understand the varied implementations frequently lumped under the label of peer review. Many programs are labeled as peer review, but often they don't use the formal, incident-based peer review that nursing needs to adopt to focus on quality of care. Understanding the other interpretations of the term, discussed later in this chapter, will help organizations understand the importance of instituting a formal, incident-based program.

Reviewing complaints about nurses

When it comes to issues of quality, nursing structures have traditionally operated as silos, keeping all information secure within their division and having little overlap with other disciplines. As issues of quality arise or complaints are made about nursing staff members, nurse leaders deal with the matter how they choose to—informally or formally.

In the informal review process, complaints can be made by the medical staff, other hospital staff, patients, families, or peers. The nursing director, and sometimes the chief nursing officer, typically reviews the complaints. The informal nature of this approach means each director deals with issues of nursing quality differently than the next. And the drawbacks are severe—individuals may be biased and not deal with every nurse or every situation in a consistent manner. In addition, issues are not always documented consistently, which may allow nurses to practice at suboptimal levels for years without notice.

Another, more formal, review process may include root cause analysis (RCA), which reduces human error through system improvements. Using this quality improvement tool allows the organization to focus on system improvements rather than individual performance, which provides an answer to the important question of what system failure caused or led to the error.

Categories of performance review

For nurses, performance evaluation typically falls into one of three categories:

1. **Pre-employment review:** The first category is the process of initially reviewing a nurse's qualifications and recommending him or her for employment after evaluating a nurse's training, experience, and current competency to perform the requested job functions.
2. **Annual performance review:** The second category of nursing performance evaluation is the annual performance review. This may include a 360-degree peer evaluation process, which looks at all aspects of the job and rates nurses' job skills and performance toward goals. (*Note:* This book does not address either the pre-employment or annual evaluation of nurses' performance.)
3. **Peer review:** The third category of evaluating nursing performance is peer review, which is the ongoing monitoring through case review and review of the nurse's work within the hospital or other healthcare settings, assessing the nurse's current competence based on nursing standards.

Most organizations do not have the sophistication to process in enough detail the level of nursing data needed to evaluate the individual nurse's performance. For example, healthcare organizations monitor The Joint Commission's National Patient Safety Goals, but few are able to identify individual nurses when there is a failure to meet the desired outcome or are able to report over time the compliance rate per nurse. Most nursing data are provided as an overall percentage of compliance by unit or floor, which is appropriate for higher-level reporting but not appropriate for evaluating an individual nursing staff member's performance based on the organization and nursing practice goals.

Developing a case review peer review program presents an opportunity both to evaluate quality of an individual nurse's work and to track and trend that data to provide a portrait over time of individual performance.

Peer review process and identifying peers

Now that we have discussed the value of peer review, it's time to tackle what the process actually entails.

Peer review is the evaluation of an individual nurse's professional practice by other nurses—that part is crucial: *evaluation by one's peers.* Peer review allows one nurse's actions to be evaluated by those who truly understand the profession and the experience of practicing at the bedside. It is not a review conducted by unfamiliar outsiders who have no experience in what they are observing.

It is the evaluation of the professional performance of individual nurses, including identification of opportunities to improve care, by an individual with the appropriate subject matter expertise to perform this evaluation.

A peer is *an individual practicing in the same profession.* The level of subject matter expertise required to provide meaningful evaluation of care will determine what practicing in the same profession means on a case-by-case basis.

As approaches to peer review have evolved, the methods for understanding how to improve patient care overall have sometimes been confused with the processes used to evaluate individual nurse performance. Both are important and are often interrelated, as they take into consideration similar things. Nevertheless, it is critical to recognize the difference between overall care improvement and the peer review process and to maintain their official separate functions. Doing so will ensure that peer review consistently and fairly evaluates each individual nurse.

Understanding the meaning of peer review

The Joint Commission describes nursing peer review as a process that is consistent, timely, defensible, balanced, and useful, with the goal of evaluating and improving nursing performance. However, as stated earlier, the term "peer review" is used interchangeably in so many contexts that some nurse professionals are confused about its true meaning. This both creates confusion and makes it hard to embrace and employ the concept.

To clear up the meaning of peer review, review the following items that are often labeled with the term but are actually other types of oversight by peers.

Some of these mislabeled items include:

- *External reviews*, such as peer review organizations (PRO) that request medical records and provide third-party oversight on the care delivered to a patient. Such PROs usually review medical necessity during hospitalization and typically do so retrospectively.
- *State nursing board peer reviews.* Some boards have formalized processes to review nurses and use peers to evaluate their quality of care, with some states having a defined process for what qualifies as a review. This is a type of peer review process, but one that is conducted by the oversight nursing body at the state level rather than direct peers.
- *Institutional review boards* (IRB). IRBs conduct reviews to ensure that appropriate clinical research protocols for the setting are followed. Although this is not considered peer review, it is an oversight function to ensure patient safety.

- *Department of Public Health (DPH) reviews.* State DPHs review patient complaints and quality-related issues. These reviews consist of an unannounced visit to the facility to review the complaint or quality concern and a chart review with interviews. This is not considered peer review but rather an oversight function.
- *Annual performance evaluations.* These are completely separate from the nursing peer review process. Nursing peer review data should be included in the overall evaluation of staff nurses' annual performance evaluation, but it is not the only data that would be used in one of these evaluations.
- *360-degree evaluations.* These are conducted by peers evaluating each other during annual performance reviews—typically on overall competencies and teamwork skills. However, they do not evaluate individual patient quality-of-care episodes and standards of practice.

These examples all differ from peer review as described in this book; here, we focus on ongoing evaluation of individual performance to identify opportunities for education and training or other actions based on the findings. This is formal, incident-based case review.

Other formal review processes

Two other important types of formal review sometimes confused with peer review are RCA and performance improvement. The common bond between them all is that they all evaluate patient care.

Root cause analysis

RCA is a form of review, but one that is much more intensive, conducted with input from a variety of disciplines, and typically done when there has been an untoward patient outcome.

RCA is the type of systems analysis required by The Joint Commission after certain types of sentinel events have occurred, such as patient death, paralysis, coma, or other permanent loss of function associated with a medical error. This multidisciplinary effort attempts to identify the causal factors that lead to variation in practice.

As such, RCA focuses primarily on systems and processes, not on individual performance. The focus progresses from special causes in clinical processes (i.e., factors that intermittently and unpredictably induce variation over and above what is inherent in the system) to common causes in organizational processes. It looks at the human and other factors most directly associated with a sentinel event and identifies risk points and their potential contributions to the event. It also either identifies potential improvements to processes or systems that would decrease the likelihood of such events happening in the future or determines, after analysis, that no such opportunities exist.

Ultimately, RCA produces an action plan that identifies the strategies healthcare organizations can use to reduce similar events in the future. Unfortunately, if the nursing peer review program is nonexistent or ineffective, the multidisciplinary RCA team may take on the task of evaluating nurse performance as well as examining the process as a whole to identify system failures. To prevent this from happening and to allow nurses to evaluate nursing practice, the best solution is to create or strengthen the nursing peer review process.

Performance improvement

Hospitals use an organization-wide approach to improve all of their processes and systems. This mechanism, called performance improvement or quality improvement, is similar to RCA in that it focuses on changing systems to improve care on an ongoing basis to meet certain standards (ideally, standards of excellence).

The performance improvement process, therefore, deals with the operations of the hospital and addresses human performance issues as an aggregate. It asks how the hospital can best train, support, and manage people to meet expectations. It does not address individual employee issues. Rather, these issues are addressed by individual employee performance evaluation and, when necessary, the hospital's disciplinary procedures.

Nursing peer review is the nurse's version of ongoing individual performance evaluation. As you will note in the following chapters, it is common during the peer review process to identify system failures that should be addressed in the overall performance improvement structure.

Nursing peer review can identify other issues that relate to organizational performance improvement in two important ways. First, in the evaluation of cases for potential nurse issues, system issues may be found that need to be addressed by the hospital's performance improvement program. Second, in evaluating individual nurse performance, it may become apparent that some issues relate closely to how care is provided by a specialty or by the medical staff as a whole. In these situations, nursing should use the hospital's performance improvement structure to best decide where the issue should be addressed.

Chapter 2

Benefits, Rationale, and Setting Clear Expectations

Learning objectives

After reading this chapter, the participant will be able to:

- List four goals of conducting peer review
- Identify the elements included in the dimensions of performance
- Describe the performance pyramid model

Historically speaking, nurses have long conducted some level of peer review: Since the first nurse conferred with another about caring for a patient, some form of peer review has been in place.

Yet when nurses are considering whether to implement a formal peer review process, or if the organization has already started down that road, many may wonder about the benefits of conducting peer review and ask questions like, "Why now?"

The Roots of Peer Review

Medical staffs have been peer reviewing their cases for decades, and as fellow professionals, we must hold ourselves to the same high standards. Nurses are professionals who must hold each other accountable and evaluate patient care so we can eliminate system and human errors. Nurses are no different than physicians in this way.

An early crusader for quality improvement, E. A. Codman helped develop the concept of outcomes management in patient care. He was a proponent of peer review and quality programs for healthcare delivered at the hospital level.

Practicing in the early 20th century, Codman was a founder of the American College of Surgeons and its Hospital Standardization Program. Eventually, that program would morph into what we know today as The Joint Commission. His statement from 1916 calling for review and transparency are as relevant today as they were a hundred years ago:

> *I am called eccentric for saying in public that hospitals, if they wish to be sure of improvement, must find out what their results are, must analyze their results to find their strong and weak points, must compare their results with those of other hospitals, must care for cases that they can care for well and avoid attempting to care for cases which they are not qualified to care for well, must welcome publicity, not only for their successes, but for their errors. Such opinions will not be eccentric a few years hence.*
>
> —*E. A. Codman, A Study in Hospital Efficiency, 1916*

Codman would likely be happy to see today that the practice of physicians reviewing the work of other physicians—peer review—is a common practice and is considered to be a crucial element of ensuring that quality medical care is provided to patients.

That element is just as crucial in the nursing profession. The major reason for implementing a peer review process is to improve patient care. If nothing else, peer review is the right thing to do to protect the patient from potential harm. It is just a matter of time before external accreditation agencies, the government, and your hospital will require a formal peer review process of nurses.

More and more, healthcare organizations are required to be transparent about quality performance metrics. While the information that is publicly reported is aggregate data, it is important for the healthcare organization to know person-specific performance data so that they can drive improved patient outcomes.

Typically, the outliers or underperformers are a small number of nurses who may not know they are not performing to the standard of care. It is important to give them specific and periodic performance feedback so that they can adjust their care model. Additionally, providing performance data to nurses helps them understand where they rank among their peers. When doing so, it is important to report the data in an anonymous way so that each nurse is uniquely identified using a coding system. This can be useful when metrics are performance based and specific in nature.

Transparency is the way of the future, and moving in that direction will help the nursing infrastructure catch up with performance models used by physicians.

The goals and benefits of peer review include:

- Improving the quality of care provided by individual nurses
- Monitoring the performance of nurses
- Identifying opportunities for performance improvement
- Identifying systemwide issues
- Identifying educational needs of nurses

If the process of peer review is to be effective, then a formal structure must be created to allow for the tracking and trending of information and the identification of potential system or human failures. Case review is useful for this, as it presents opportunities to identify failures through investigation so nurses and other team members can correct them before injury occurs in another patient or patients.

The Nursing Performance Pyramid

Organizations do not achieve outstanding results by accident—they take a powerful, common-sense approach that motivates all employees to consistently do their best.

The Walt Disney Company is a fantastic example of a company that takes such an approach to motivating employees and thus ensures that every single staff member in its theme parks is uniformly nice, upbeat, and helpful, whether that staff member is the person in the concession stand or the ticket taker or the person dressed up as Mickey Mouse. Other companies that understand and apply this process to provide outstanding service day in and day out are luxury hotels, such as The Ritz-Carlton.

These exceptional organizations apply an approach that promotes outstanding individual performance, called the *performance pyramid*. At its core, the power of the pyramid is a human resource management tool. It has been taught for years by the American College of Physician Executives, who successfully pioneered applying this model to hospital medical staffs. Now is the time to apply the same model to nurses.

FIGURE 2.1 **The power of the pyramid—Achieving great nurse performance**

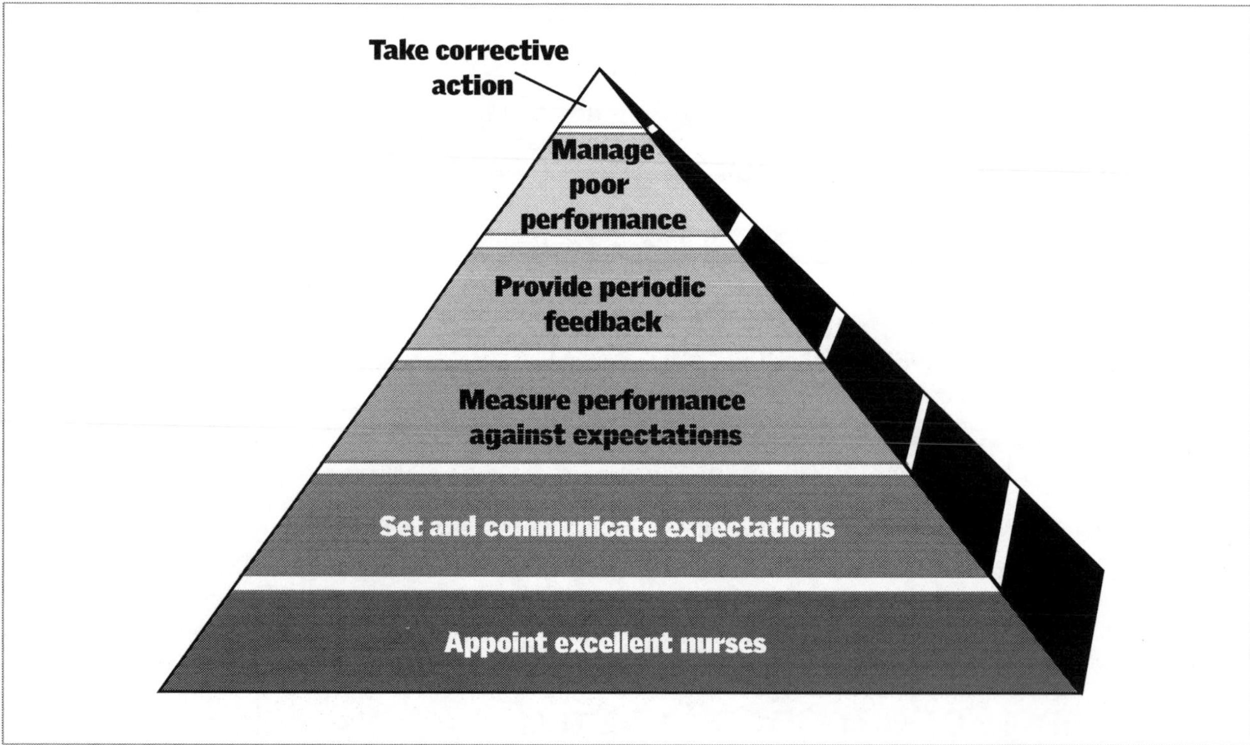

Figure 2.1 illustrates the performance pyramid model, which is outlined in the rest of this chapter. The performance pyramid model is a common-sense approach to creating a nursing performance improvement culture.

As you can see, the pyramid is built in layers. Each layer represents an essential responsibility that nursing leaders must carry out to optimize nurse performance. The model is designed in the shape of a pyramid because the more time leaders spend on the base layers, the less time they will have to spend on the upper layers, especially the disruptive and challenging tasks of managing poor performance and taking corrective action.

Let's take a look at the six layers of the pyramid and the role of each in improving nurse performance.

Appoint excellent nurses

If you start by bringing nursing staff into the hospital who are well qualified and competent, you improve your ability to reach the level of excellence you desire. For example, consider Disney Company employees. Why are they so polite and friendly? It isn't simply because Disney trains them to be, but rather because the company carefully seeks out people who have these attributes in the first place. Thus, careful selection is the essence of the first layer of the pyramid.

Carefully selecting nurses requires solid screening systems. When a nurse first applies for a staff position, his or her professional credentials (e.g., licensure, education, experience, current competence) must be verified in accordance with policy and procedure, state and federal regulations, and accreditation standards (e.g., The Joint Commission or the National Committee for Quality Assurance).

This is the point where it is crucial to go beyond minimum requirements—*do not stop here.* Create and maintain the highest possible standard for nursing. For example, require applicants for positions in your facility to demonstrate excellent previous clinical performance, provide superior professional references, and demonstrate the ability to relate well to colleagues and other employees.

Set and communicate expectations

Few organizations take the time to define and explain in one document what is expected of a nurse on staff in the organization. Despite the importance of doing so, nursing departments often do not set and communicate expectations well. Normally, job descriptions describe job functions and requirements but often fail in describing nursing expectations. For example, a job description may describe the qualification such as educational level but not describe the technical quality of care expected of the nurse.

The nursing department should communicate to every new nurse, in writing, what is expected of him or her to achieve excellence. This is your opportunity to establish expectations for the type of nursing culture you want. In a document you will provide to each new nurse, define the routines and protocols that are used and acceptable in the organization.

Consider it a statement of the culture of the nursing staff, including information about professionalism and the standards of nursing practice. You can view it as a kind of executive summary of the organization's policies and procedures. At the minimum, the document should outline the essential dimensions of nursing performance:

- Technical quality of care
- Patient safety and rights
- Quality of service
- Resource utilization
- Peer-to-peer relationships

Figure 2.2 shows a partial example of this type of document. The full document is available in the download section of this book.

FIGURE 2.2 | **Sample nurse expectations statement**

Nursing Expectations

The expectations described in this document reflect current nursing governance bylaws and hospital policies and procedures. This document is designed to bring together the most important issues found in those documents, along with some key concepts that reflect our nursing culture, vision, and standards of practice.

Nursing leaders will work to improve individual and aggregate nursing performance through nonpunitive approaches and providing appropriate positive and negative feedback that allows each nurse the opportunity to grow and develop in his or her capabilities to provide outstanding patient care and make valuable contributions to our hospital and community.

Technical quality of care

- Achieve nursing outcomes that consistently meet or exceed generally accepted clinical standards for the nursing discipline
- Provide nursing care based upon the generally accepted clinical nursing standards and hospital policy

Patient safety/patient rights

- Participate in hospital efforts to reduce adverse patient care events
- Protect patient information based on hospital policy/government regulations and ensure that information is kept confidential
- Communicate all pertinent patient information to other members of the healthcare team
- Communicate effectively with patients and their families regarding nursing interventions and care
- Provide emotional and physical support to patients and families
- Provide comfort to patients, including prompt and effective nursing management
- Wear hospital identification at all times

Quality of service

- Provide timely and continuous nursing care of patients
- Maintain medical records consistent with the hospital policies, including, but not limited to, chart entry legibility and timely completion of initial nursing assessment, care plans, and notes

FIGURE 2.2 | **Sample nurse expectations statement (cont'd.)**

- When calling the attending physician, provide adequate communication regarding patient care needs, nursing interventions, and outcomes using the SBAR communication format:
  - Situation
  - Background
  - Assessment
  - Recommendation
- Support nursing leaders' and staff members' efforts to exceed patient satisfaction rates for nursing units

Resource utilization

- Strive to provide quality patient care that is cost-effective by cooperating with efforts to appropriately manage the use of valuable patient care resources
- Ensure patient care testing is scheduled when ordered and is timely
- Provide timely discharge instructions in collaboration with other caregivers

Peer and coworker relationships

- At all times, act in a professional, respectful manner with patients, physicians, other nurses, administrators, board members, and other hospital personnel to enhance a spirit of cooperation and mutual respect and trust among members of the patient care team
- Refrain from inappropriate behavior, as outlined in the "employee code of conduct" policy toward members of the hospital and medical staff, patients, or their families
- Refrain from documentation in the medical record that does not directly relate to the clinical status of the patient and plan of care or that is derogatory or inflammatory concerning the care provided to the patient

Contributions to hospital and community

- Participate, if requested, in relevant quality improvement activities or community services
- Support actions and decisions in accordance with the hospital's mission statement and strategic plan
- Review your individual and specialty data for all dimensions of performance and utilize these data to continuously improve care

Contributions to hospital and community

Nurses must know that these are the expectations that the organization sets for them as employees, and they should know that these are the expectations nurses should have of each other. Before you start the peer review process, it is beneficial to sit down with nursing leaders and future peer review committee members to define what is expected of the organization's nurses.

Once the document has been created, it should be shared with currently employed nurses, and each new member of your team should be presented with a copy of this document during the orientation process.

If expectations have not been clearly established, you will find that each staff nurse you talk to has a different perception of what is expected of staff. Sometimes, this is a result of information overload. How can we expect nurses to know the hundreds of policies within the organization?

Consider, for example, what happens when a nurse admits a patient and must complete the nursing assessment within 24 hours of admission. One nurse completes the entire assessment—every line. Another nurse fills in some of the assessment, doesn't enter comments, and leaves blanks in a few areas, despite the fact that comments are required to consider the assessment complete. Is this appropriate? Why does one nurse complete every detail and the other leaves blanks and thinks it is acceptable?

Consider also the nurse who is working with a scoring algorithm that reveals that a patient needs a nutritional referral. The nurse checks that a referral is needed but never issues the referral to the nutritionist because the nurse does not know it is her or his responsibility.

Setting expectations and holding nurses accountable are crucial. Review current policies and reinforce cultural values. Although expectations vary from organization to organization, the tools can be used as an example for setting expectations of staff nurses.

Measure performance against expectations

The basic premise of any successful quality program is that measuring something drives improvement, an idea embodied in the saying "If you can't measure it, you can't manage it."

Once a hospital has established expectations and communicated them to the nursing staff, it must measure each nurse's performance against those expectations and immediately decide how often to monitor nursing documentation for key elements in the medical record.

The answer, of course, is continuously. And the result of that monitoring is always the same: We always have deficiencies. But without detailed information, how can we determine who has the deficiencies and why?

More often than not, we monitor nurses using the percentage of compliance to evaluate nursing care. For example, we find that there is a 45% deficiency rate in completing the nursing assessment within 24 hours of admission, which is hospital policy. But using just one percentage rate-based indicator penalizes the nurses who always meet our expectations, while allowing the other nurses to slip through the cracks and not be noticed. We may assume nurses need more training and further reiteration of the policy, when actually it may only be a few nurses who are noncompliant with the hospital policy—and they are responsible for bringing the percentage down. Nurses responsible for the deficiency never meet our benchmarks or goals, and we do not know who they are, so we can't ask why.

Therefore, once nursing indicators are established, you will take your quality program to the next level by identifying each individual's performance. The insights you gain will provide you with a genuinely useful tool for improvement.

NOTE › Before instituting individual performance monitoring, nursing leaders must ensure that all nurses know that their performance will be measured, how it will be measured, and how it will be compared to that of their peers.

Provide periodic feedback

Individuals can't possibly know whether or not they are meeting expectations unless they receive periodic feedback about their performance. The typical annual evaluation is not enough—feedback must be frequent and targeted.

Providing nurses with frequent feedback on their performance is essential and reinforces the expectations established by the organization. When nurses receive constructive feedback in a timely and easy-to-follow-manner, they will use it for self-improvement.

Equally important is to provide nurses with detailed feedback and appreciation when they perform well, not just when they perform poorly. Remember, the goal is not to weed out the bad apples but rather to give each individual nurse every opportunity to improve and excel, in order to provide quality, safe patient care.

Manage poor performance

Nursing leaders should address performance issues as they are documented. Discuss such issues with the appropriate nurse as soon as concerns arise. For example, if a feedback report shows that a nurse is not meeting performance expectations and the nurse does not self-correct, appropriate leaders or mentors (if your organization has a mentoring program) should meet with the nurse to discuss improvement strategies. Leaders and mentors can help motivate the nurse to change or eliminate unacceptable performance by following these jointly developed strategies. They can provide useful advice and direction for doing so and should monitor the nurse's progress.

This layer of the pyramid is the most uncomfortable for nurse leaders who have not been trained to manage poor performance collegially and effectively, but avoiding performance issues is unfair to nurses and dangerous to patients. Without proper training, nurse leaders often avoid such confrontations because they are difficult, and situations are left unaddressed until seriously negative data forces leaders to act.

Note that managing poor performance is not the same as taking corrective action, which should help nurse leaders feel more comfortable with this role. Rather, managing poor performance consists of a series of well-designed and well-executed interventions designed to help the nurse improve. As noted earlier, constructive ongoing nursing feedback is essential, so hopefully this step is avoided. The first of these interventions should be collegial and follow the hospital's disciplinary action process.

If the nurse does not improve following an initial intervention, ensuing interventions progress according to hospital policy—but remember that the goal of all such interventions is to help the nurse be the best nurse she or he can be.

Take corrective action

Nursing leadership must act when all of the steps outlined in this chapter have been taken, yet the nurse fails to self-improve and her or his poor performance threatens quality and safety of the patient. Such action is known as corrective action and is a formal process that involves progressive discipline, with the possibility of the extreme action of termination.

> **CAUTION >** Nursing leaders must consult HR or the appropriate authority before corrective action is taken.

Applying the Pyramid to Nursing Culture

Success in providing patient quality care occurs with a combination of the right people, the right equipment, the right processes, and the right culture. The same is true for peer review.

In this chapter, we've provided a description of what the right culture should look like. The remaining chapters will address the legal framework, the right equipment (structure and tools), and the right process (procedures and methods) you will need to create a contemporary and useful peer review program that improves nurse performance and improves patient outcomes.

Chapter 3

Immunity, Confidentiality, and Protecting Information From Discovery

Learning objectives

After reading this chapter, the participant will be able to:

- Describe the three types of peer review protection laws
- Describe the components of the Health Care Quality and Improvement Act of 1986
- Name two ways of protecting peer review information

When contemplating establishing a peer review process, many healthcare organizations worry about the legal and confidential aspects. Is peer review protected? If nurse reviewers discuss a case, could they find themselves in court giving evidence if a plaintiff decides to sue? These are all valid concerns and must be addressed before the process is begun.

Peer Review Protection Laws

Before establishing your peer review process, you must familiarize yourself with the following three categories of peer review protection laws:

1. **Immunity related:** Those granting immunity from lawsuits to persons and institutions. "A professional review action must meet the standards set forth in the Healthcare Quality and Improvement Act in order to qualify for immunity. The professional review action must be taken:

a. In the reasonable belief that the action was in furtherance of quality healthcare

b. After a reasonable effort to obtain the facts of the matter

c. After adequate notice and hearing procedures afforded to physician or other such procedures that are fair to the physician

d. In the reasonable belief that the action was warranted by the facts known after the reasonable effort to obtain the facts and adequate notice and hearing procedures have been afforded to the clinician" *(www.healthlawyers.org/hlresources/Health%20Law%20Wiki/HCQIA.aspx)*

2. **Privilege related:** Those declaring peer review work products to be privileged and inadmissible in court. An example of this would be nursing case (peer) review completed forms evaluating a nurse's care. The form is protected and will not be produced for a lawsuit.

3. **Confidentiality related:** Those allowing information related to peer review to remain confidential. Any documents or actions taken as a result of peer review are confidential and thus protected from being produced in a court of law.

These laws affect lawsuits brought by plaintiffs. As you know, most malpractice lawsuits are brought against the physician and the "deep pocket" or hospital, naming all of those who had significant impact in the care of the patient and outcome.

Lawsuits against nurses typically stem from that deep-pocket strategy; in today's climate, nurses often are named in the lawsuit. Rarely, however, is a nurse the only target of a medical malpractice lawsuit, because the plaintiff will want to target the physician who is responsible for the care as well as the hospital so that more damages can be filed, increasing the size of the award.

In fact, a patient who is suing may name the same deep-pocket defendants or hospital and request related peer review information to support a malpractice claim. Remember that peer review statutes do not actually prevent a plaintiff from filing a lawsuit. Basically, anybody who has enough money to pay filing fees can file a lawsuit. Although the suit may be dismissed immediately, it still will have been filed, which can be very distressing for anyone named in it. Being named in a lawsuit is traumatic and can cause good competent staff to become disillusioned with the medical industry.

Professional liability coverage

Nurse peer reviewers should note that a hospital's insurance policy typically covers all good-faith peer review participants and, thus, would cover any suits filed, even frivolous ones. Coverage includes providing a legal defense for individually named nurse peer reviewers and coverage in the event that monetary damages are assessed, which is almost never.

Hospital professional liability policies also provide some coverage to protect peer review information from discoverability, but it would be best to review with legal counsel the protection and coverage in your state.

Immunity

Immunity addresses the nurse's and hospital's fears that they could be found liable for significant monetary damages in defamation or negligent lawsuits. The federal government and all state governments have passed immunity statutes of some kind.

The Health Care Quality and Improvement Act of 1986

The federal Health Care Quality and Improvement Act of 1986 (HCQIA) grants immunity to healthcare professionals who engage in good-faith evaluation of their peers. To qualify for federal immunity, however, the peer review decision must be a professional review with action taken by a professional review body. The HCQIA defines a professional review action as "an action or recommendation of a professional review body which is taken or made in the conduct of a professional review activity which is based on the competence or professional conduct of an individual."

The HCQIA defines a professional review body as a "committee of a health care entity which conducts professional review activity, and includes any committee assisting the governing body in a professional review activity." This act was introduced to address two longstanding practitioner problems: practitioners being reluctant to engage in peer review and incompetent practitioners moving from state to state without a record.

State immunity laws

The majority of state statutes provide peer reviewers immunity from civil liability. The strongest statutes give immunity to all peer review committee members and the institutions and persons furnishing information to it; weaker statutes give immunity for only a few or specified people. Not that the immunity is absolute—as with HCQIA, most states have qualified their grant of immunity. Many require the peer review action to have been taken without malice or in good faith.

Privilege: Protection From Discovery

The second type of protection is the work product privilege, which prevents information associated with the peer review process from being discovered. This protection is based on the idea that nurses will not candidly discuss a colleague's shortcoming if their statements later could be discovered in judicial proceedings. All of the states, as well as the District of Columbia, recognize some form of privilege that protects various records and documents created as a part of the peer review process. HCQIA does not protect peer review documents from federal discovery.

State laws vary regarding which documents are considered protected, so it is wise to understand your state statutes before implementing this process so that you can incorporate additional safety measures as needed.

Privilege guidelines

This entire peer review process is part of the hospital's peer review program and structure. Discuss with legal counsel how to further protect the information under the hospital's current peer review policy and state statutes. In addition, consult with legal counsel to ensure that this language and policy are in parallel with other institutional policies.

Language specifying the confidential nature of this information is critical. The following policies should be reflected in the appropriate document:

1. The contents of the peer evaluation files remain the sole property of the hospital and may not be examined by any outside agency, client, patient, or legal authority. Once the information is given outside of the protected internal peer review structure, it could become discoverable. Discoverability means that the information is outside the protected peer review structure and available to the plaintiff's attorney. For example, if copies of a case review form are sent to a concerned family member, that family member (or the patient) is not considered within the peer review confines of the hospital. No copies should ever be made or distributed outside the peer review structure within the hospital.
2. Each member of the nursing peer review committee and any persons consulted by the committee will be instructed by the committee chairperson about his or her responsibility to protect the confidentiality of information. This applies both to patient information and to the proceedings of the committee. Each committee member and anyone interviewed will read and sign the peer review confidentiality guidelines form (which is included as Figure 4.5 in Chapter 4). The confidentiality statement should be signed annually by everyone on the committee, even if you have the same representatives from the previous year.

The confidentiality statement should also be signed by any new member who is appointed to the committee. These confidentiality statements should be archived in a secure location.

3. The committee shall keep its information, opinions, and proceedings entirely confidential, except that the committee shall disclose on request written or oral communication made to the committee and the records and proceedings of the committee, with the approval of the chairperson/CEO, to:
   a. Law enforcement authorities investigating a criminal matter
   b. The state board of registration or licenser of any state
   c. Another professional nursing peer review committee or a state board of nursing–approved peer assistance program
   d. Appropriate state or federal agencies

Confidentiality: Security of Information

All peer review information is privileged and confidential in accordance with nursing and hospital bylaws, state and federal laws, and regulations pertaining to confidentiality and nondiscoverability.

To further protect the information, the following procedures should be implemented:

1. The hospital will keep nurse-specific peer review and other quality information concerning a nurse in a secure, locked file archived in nursing administration. The peer review and quality information will be kept separate from the employment file. Nurse-specific peer review information consists of information related to:
   a. Performance data for all dimensions of performance measured for that individual nurse
   b. The individual nurse's role in sentinel events, significant incidents, or near misses
   c. Correspondence to the nurse regarding commendations, comments regarding practice performance, or corrective action taken
2. Peer review information is available only to authorized individuals who have a legitimate need to know this information based upon their responsibilities as nursing leaders or hospital employees. However, they shall have access to the information only to the extent necessary to carry out their assigned responsibilities. Only the following individuals shall have access to nurse-specific peer review information and only for purposes of quality improvement:
   a. Vice president, nursing
   b. Administrative director, nursing operations

c. Individuals surveying for accrediting bodies with appropriate jurisdiction (e.g., The Joint Commission or state/federal regulatory bodies)

d. Individuals with a legitimate purpose for access as determined by the hospital board of directors

3. No copies of peer review documents will be created and distributed unless authorized by the vice president of nursing or per hospital policy.

CAUTION > If ever in question, it is best to consult legal counsel for advice.

Chapter 4

STEP 1

Designing a Formal Structure to Support the Peer Review Process

Learning objectives

After reading this chapter, the participant will be able to:

- Describe the advantages of using a formalized, rather than informal, structure to support peer review
- Identify three goals of the nursing peer review committee

Once your organization has decided to adopt a formal case review system, the first step in creating it is deciding how the program will be structured and how it will look at your facility. The rest of this book will walk you through all the steps you need to begin your program.

Functions of Peer Review

The peer review structure you create must be able to accommodate two functions: evaluation and oversight. The first function, evaluation, is the familiar process of actually evaluating a nurse's performance. The second function, oversight, is less familiar and can create confusion.

The oversight function involves all the actions necessary to oversee the process and ensure that it is done correctly. This includes creating policy, establishing a charter, and deciding how to keep track of the information and data created over time.

As noted in Chapter 1, the data that can be collected are often new for nursing; it is important for the profession to move toward a formal structure so that this important information is not lost.

As you can imagine, informal structures typically do not document information on an ongoing basis, and thus the data serve no useful purpose. Losing valuable information or not using that information may affect patient care; therefore, it is crucial to create a formal structure that can track and then trend this data over time.

The formal peer review process can support each of these two functions.

Identify a Formal Structure That Works for You

One structure does not prevail when incorporating nursing peer review; there are many ways to proceed. It is important to remember to keep it simple, and one way to do that is to integrate the functions into an existing committee if possible. Most existing nursing structures will easily accommodate integration of this process.

Some organizations make the mistake of creating an additional committee for the sole purpose of peer review, when staff are already overwhelmed with responsibilities and feel that they are spending less time with patients.

Shared governance structure

Incorporating peer review into your organization's shared governance structure is relatively simple, because a formal framework is already in place. Review your shared governance structure and determine where the quality or peer review council would fit. For example, it may fit best under the nurse practice council. In some instances, the nursing peer review process and committee may fit most appropriately under the realm of a hospital quality oversight committee or under the medical staff quality committee.

Take a look at Figure 4.1, which provides an example of a nursing shared governance structure.

The oversight function and reporting obligations

Many facilities do not have well-organized quality oversight in nursing. The oversight function can also become an afterthought in the peer review process, conducted only when the quality staff asks for guidance to resolve cases that are deemed beyond appropriate.

To create an evaluation process that truly focuses on nurse performance, the nursing staff must establish an active oversight structure with clearly assigned responsibilities that support the goals of peer review. Such an oversight structure will, for example, make informed case determinations, select relevant nursing measures for performance dimensions, and prioritize resource use.

FIGURE 4.1 **Nursing shared governance structure**

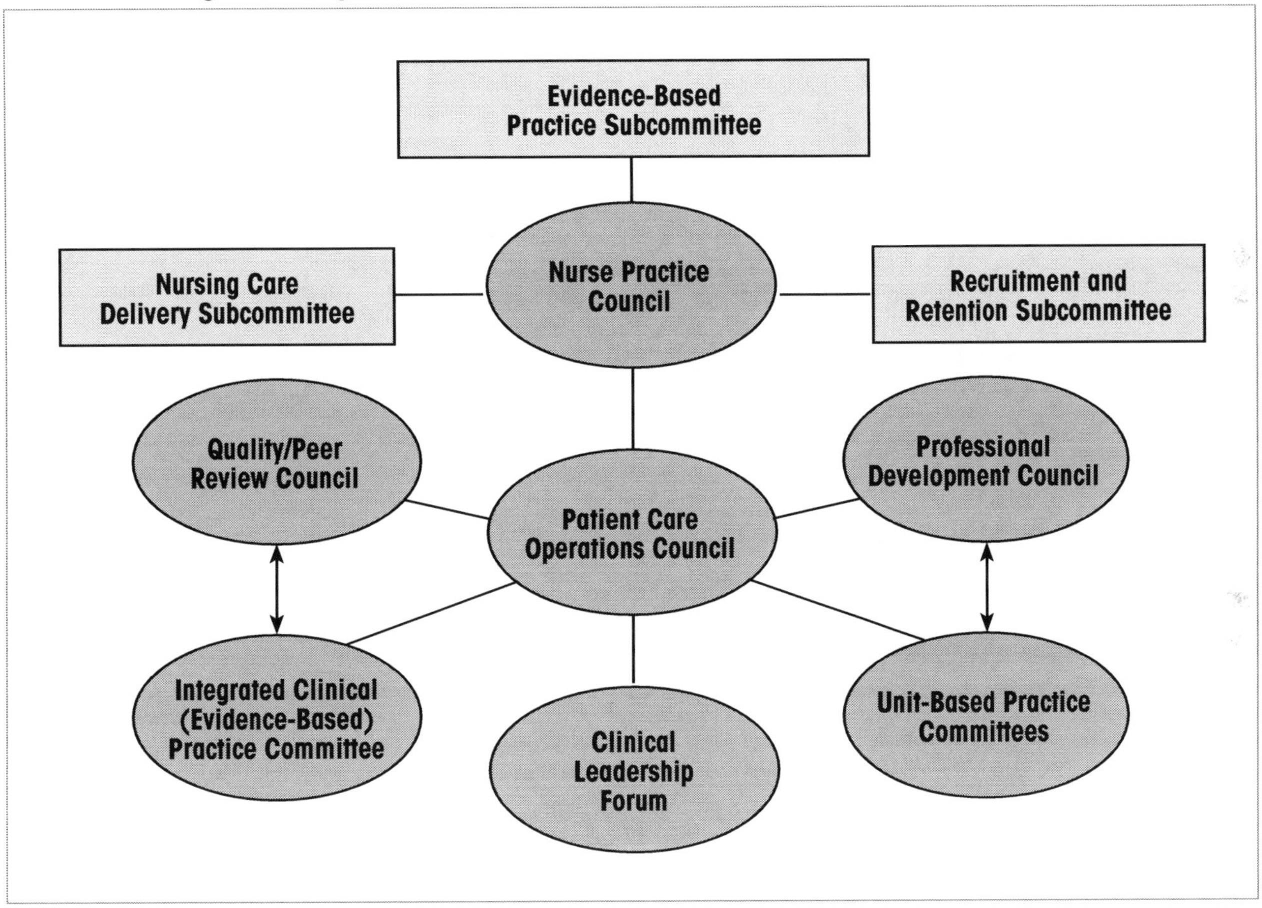

Oversight within a shared governance structure

As illustrated in Figure 4.2, developing a committee reporting process defines where and what kind of information will be reported and to which committee. The reporting diagram in this case would be used in a shared governance model.

FIGURE 4.2 **Nursing peer review shared governance reporting structure**

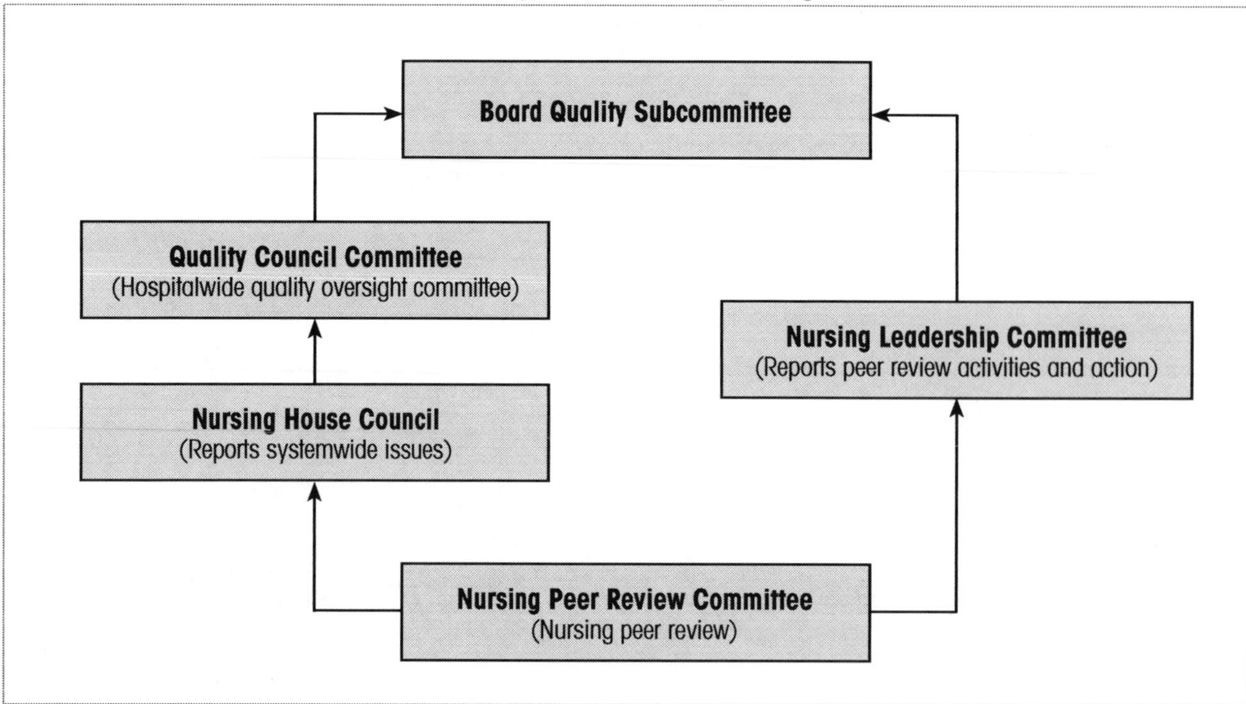

In this example, the oversight information is reported in the following manner:

1. **Nursing peer review responsibilities are conducted within the nursing peer review committee who reports to the:**
   - *Nursing leadership committee.* The information reported to this committee provides leadership with enough detailed information to take action if necessary and to guide the nursing peer review committee chair in certain circumstances. In this forum, nursing leadership should know the outcome of each case reviewed and recommendations from the nursing peer review committee.
   - *Nursing house council.* The council should evaluate all hospital-wide nursing issues identified during case review. Such issues might include policy development, identification of nursing process failure, or educational needs. Only the final determinations of the case and action/follow-up would be reported to this council.
2. **The nursing house council will report nursing issues and resolutions to the hospital-wide quality oversight committee,** whose responsibility it is to provide oversight for all quality issues within the organization and report to the board quality subcommittee, which should receive all high-level information pertaining to nursing quality and improvements.

NOTE > When discussing peer review activities, it is important to protect peer review information based on regulatory and accreditation program requirements and state laws. More detail regarding legal protection and confidentiality of information can be found in Chapter 3.

Other nursing structures

If you don't already have a shared governance structure, do not feel that you need to create one simply to introduce peer review. Many other nursing structures work just as well; we don't recommend that you change your current structure to a shared governance model simply to incorporate peer review. If you try to undertake too many changes simultaneously, you will find the process becoming difficult to manage, which could result in failure to establish an effective peer review process.

If your nursing structure is limited, then your final option is to create a new committee simply to focus on peer review. One option to consider is to create a nursing peer review process that assimilates an existing medical staff peer review process. We don't recommend that you incorporate peer review into an existing nursing management committee—the nurses will inevitably feel that this is a punitive process.

NOTE > More detail regarding suggested membership of the committee is located in the peer review charter (Figure 4.4).

Oversight without a shared governance structure

The structure shown in Figure 4.3 is for organizations that don't have a shared governance model. The same reporting process holds true for this structure, in that the nursing peer review committee has an obligation to report systemwide issues to the hospital quality committee and specific peer review activities and action to nursing leadership.

Ultimately, the board has responsibility for ensuring quality and therefore should have a quarterly report of activities.

FIGURE 4.3 **Nursing peer review reporting structure**

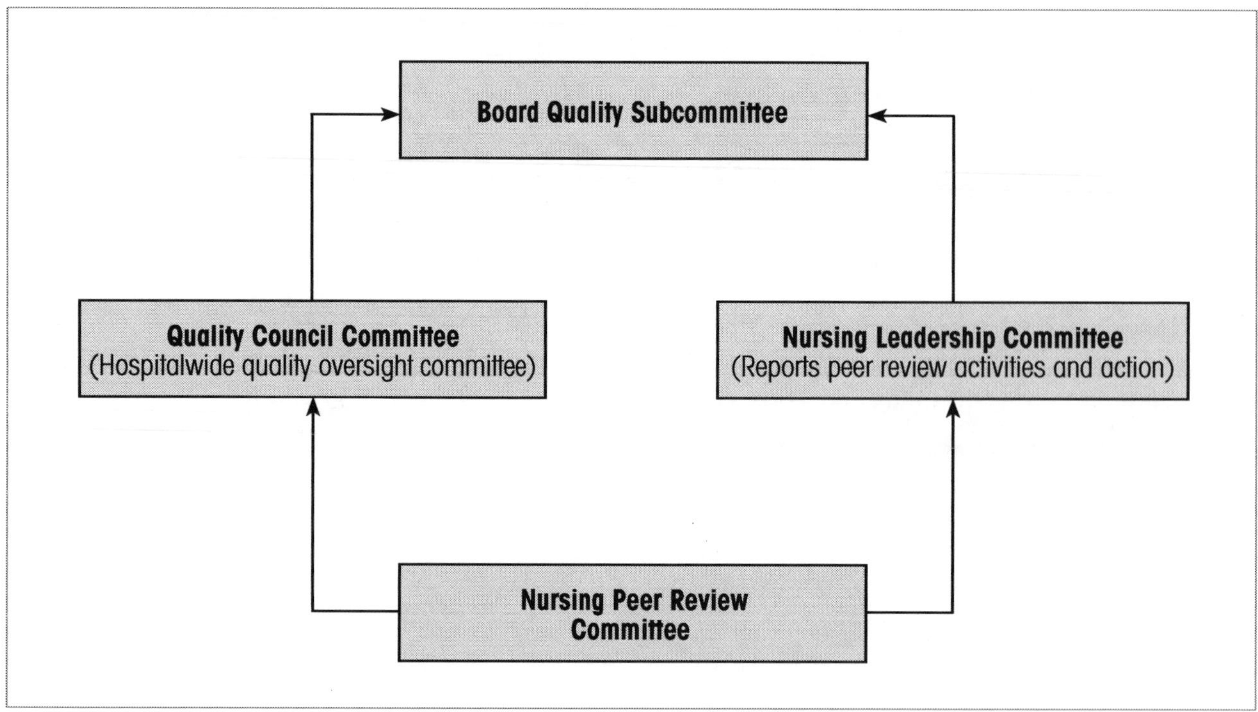

Defining Committee Roles and Responsibilities

After you have chosen how to fit peer review into the nursing structure, the next step is to decide how a committee will be structured and what it will do. We recommend that you create some form of committee charter to define the goals, scope, responsibilities, membership, frequency of meetings, and reporting obligations. Once a charter has been developed, it can guide committee members and answer staff questions regarding committee functions.

See Figure 4.4 for a sample nursing peer review committee charter you can adapt for your own facility. The charter is the place where you should identify for everyone the goals of the committee. It is imperative to outline the scope and responsibilities of the committee so it will handle only appropriate cases and so it concerns itself only with issues for which it was designed.

The charter also allows you to publicize how cases can be referred to peer review, as well as such basic housekeeping issues as who will comprise the membership and when the committee will meet.

FIGURE 4.4 **Sample nursing peer review committee charter**

Nursing Peer Review Committee Charter

Goals

To establish a centralized, multispecialty approach for the nursing staff to improve nursing performance on an individual and aggregate level, your facility accomplishes the following goals:

1. Improve patient outcomes
2. Enhance nursing performance
3. Increase efficiency of the process for the nursing staff
4. Identify system/process barriers impacting patient care
5. Maintain nursing department educational goals
6. Improve use of support resources

Scope

The nursing peer review committee will be responsible for evaluating all areas of nursing competency and improving nursing performance in the areas of clinical quality, patient safety, nursing responsiveness, and documentation issues.

Responsibilities

Individual nursing case review

- Perform initial nurse review of all cases identified by referral or using the approved screening criteria. Obtain reviews and recommendations from nursing clinical experts when required.
- Communicate with the nurse involved in the case to obtain input prior to making determinations when opportunities for improvement may exist.
- Make determinations regarding opportunities for individual or system improvements based on individual case review.

Use of rate and rule indicators

- Perform regular review for individual outliers from nursing staff rule or rate indicator data for all nurse competencies within the nursing charter scope. This function may be delegated by the nursing chair or to an individual nursing peer review member.

FIGURE 4.4 | **Sample nursing peer review committee charter (cont'd.)**

- Identify potential individual nursing opportunities for improvement or determine whether further evaluation is needed to define whether an improvement opportunity exists.
- Identify potential nursing staff opportunities for improvement.
- Identify potential medical practice or hospital system opportunities for improvement.
- Make final determinations regarding opportunities for individual or system improvements based on the results of rate or rule indicators.

Improvement opportunities

Addressing improvement opportunities will be the role of the house quality oversight committee and nursing leadership. The role of the nursing peer review committee is to ensure that, when opportunities for improvement are identified, the appropriate individuals are notified of the issues and a reasonable improvement plan is developed. This will be accomplished through the following:

- Communicate individual improvement opportunities to nursing leadership, who develop an improvement plan if necessary
- Communicate system improvement opportunities to the hospital quality oversight committee
- The support staff will track responses and improvement plans
- Review the improvement plan
- Report to the appropriate committee regularly regarding actions taken to improve care and any cases where action was not taken when requested or actions are perceived to be inadequate

Performance improvement system management

- Approve requests to the quality management department for additions or deletions to indicators, criteria, or focused studies for evaluating nursing performance
- At least annually, review the indicators, screening tools, and referral systems for effectiveness in collaboration with the nursing staff and recommend changes to nursing leadership

FIGURE 4.4 | **Sample nursing peer review committee charter (cont'd.)**

The following areas are considered outside the committee's scope:

1. Individual nursing performance issues regarding nursing behavior will be the responsibility of nursing leadership.
2. Medical staff or systems issues identified during the course of a review. The appropriate committee(s) should be notified for further review and/or follow-up.

Membership

The membership will comprise members from maternal child services, surgical services, inpatient services, and critical services. The chair of the committee and members will be appointed by the chief nursing officer.

Meetings

The committee will meet monthly. The presence of five voting committee members will constitute a quorum during a regularly scheduled meeting for the purposes of making case determinations.

Reporting

The committee will report monthly to the hospital quality oversight committee on non-peer review activities (system improvements) and to nursing leadership on peer review activities and action.

Committee members

The sample peer review committee charter recommends that peer review committee members be appointed by nursing leadership. Nursing leadership may take recommendations from people such as the president of the shared governance council.

Identifying members for the committee is an important function and one that sometimes causes concern, but the three key elements ensure that high-quality committee members will be appointed:

1. **Membership is composed solely of nursing staff.** However, more modern structures may invite a member of the medical staff peer review committee to be a representative who is a nonvoting member on the committee. A medical staff representative helps foster open communication between the medical and nursing peer review committees. If nursing issues

are identified during medical staff peer review, then the physician representative can report these issues to the nursing committee. Likewise, if physician issues are identified during nursing case review, then the physician representative will report back to the medical staff peer review. For example, an issue that might be identified is the case of a nurse attempting to call a physician regarding a patient's condition but receiving no response from him or her. This should be reviewed by the medical staff. It can also be useful in the review process to include a physician who can assist in answering questions related to diagnosis or treatment protocols.

2. **Membership should include representatives from your organization's most prominent service lines who have sound clinical judgment and skills.** Most of the cases reviewed by the committee will involve the larger service lines, merely due to patient volume, and the high-risk areas, such as the emergency department and intensive care units. Having representatives from these service lines will ensure knowledgeable members who are familiar with patient care protocols in these areas.

3. **Membership should be composed of unbiased individuals who have the ability to be objective during case review and who are not quick to render judgment.** These individuals are likely seasoned nurses who have at least a few years of patient care experience. They should also be respected members of the organization who are recognized as leaders on their units and as excellent clinicians.

In addition, membership can include a non-clinical administrative individual to support the committee with case generation and assignment, creation of meeting agendas, and completion of committee meeting minutes and reports.

Impartiality

When appointing committee members, it is important to identify unbiased nurses who can act professionally and take the responsibility seriously. The committee members must be impartial in their decisions.

In this country, the United States Constitution guarantees us the right to trial by jury, not the right to a jury of our peers. What the Sixth Amendment grants us is the right to an impartial jury—and the adjective "impartial" is key to determining who should serve as a peer. Like the members of a jury, a nurse peer reviewer should be as objective and impartial as possible.

A commitment to impartiality is key to receiving buy-in from the nursing staff about the whole peer review process. By selecting nurse reviewers who are known to be fair-minded and objective, you underscore that the committee is impartial.

In an ideal world, you would be able to select peer reviewers who have no arguable bias in favor of or against each nurse whose care is being evaluated. However, in the real world, individual bias can never be completely eliminated. The effects of any bias can be reduced by ensuring that it is the peer review committee, rather than any one nurse peer reviewer, that makes the ultimate decisions. This fact should be communicated to nursing staff so that they understand the committee is a cohesive whole not dominated by any one interest.

Conflict of interest

Related to impartiality is conflict of interest. Conflict of interest refers to situations in which financial or other personal considerations may adversely affect, or simply have the appearance of adversely affecting, a committee member's professional judgment about a nurse or a situation and therefore affect their ability to exercise impartiality in their responsibilities.

Prior to convening the committee, you should establish that any nurse reviewer with a potential conflict of interest is ethically obligated to disclose it to the rest of the peer review committee. The committee can then determine whether the conflict is substantial enough that the peer reviewer should be excluded from decision-making about this case.

The determination of conflict of interest will always be a judgment call, and the committee will need to decide on a case-by-case basis. The only absolute conflict of interest that can be clearly stated beforehand is when the issue or issues in the case directly involves the reviewer or a committee member. Just as judges who have a personal interest in cases must recuse themselves to avoid even the appearance of impropriety, peer reviewers should excuse themselves in such situations.

Most conflict-of-interest situations, however, are not that clear—they are usually relative. Two actions are necessary to resolve conflicts of interest so that, should a judge or jury examine the situation from the outside, there will be no doubt as to whether the peer review was conducted in good faith.

- First, all nurses who serve on the peer review committee must be scrupulously honest about disclosing potential conflicts of interest, including relevant personal issues to the other members of the committee. For example, one such issue may be that a nurse under peer review is engaged in a bitter divorce with a committee member's brother.
- Second, the peer review committee itself must use its judgment and combined wisdom to determine whether a particular nurse can render a reasonably objective opinion. This judgment may be based both on the nurse's reputation for fairness and on the nature and intensity of the conflict. If the committee has doubts, it should always err on the side of safety and either assign a different reviewer or obtain an external review.

Set and Communicate Nursing Expectations

Once the committee structure has been determined and the charter written, it is crucial to help participants understand what is expected of them as peer review committee members.

As discussed in Chapter 2, few organizations have taken the time to define in one document what is expected of a nurse on staff in their organization. But doing so is worth the time, and you can use Figure 2.2 to create your own expectations.

This one-page document states the culture of the nursing staff—"how we do things here"—and acts as a kind of executive summary of policies and procedures. The document will help new committee members understand both their own responsibilities and the standards to which they will hold those whom they review.

Protecting Confidential Information

Before any further steps can be taken and the process begun, it is vital to establish a way to protect confidential information.

Protecting the confidential and extremely sensitive information that will be covered in peer review is essential at the start of your review process. Committee members need to be educated about the importance of keeping all information confidential and never discussing it with anyone outside the confines of the peer review committee.

To further reiterate the importance of confidentiality, have all committee members sign a statement each year that they will keep the proceedings confidential. Figure 4.5 is an example of confidential guidelines that can be signed by each committee member and archived with the committee minutes in a locked and secure area.

NOTE > It is important to have each member sign a copy each year so they remember the guidelines for dealing with confidential information. In addition, new members must sign a copy when they join the committee.

Figure 4.5 can be adapted to suit your organization's needs. It may be necessary to add language to reflect your state's peer review requirements or to increase protection of confidential peer review information from discovery. Once again, if you are unsure of state requirements, consult legal experts for guidance.

FIGURE 4.5 | **Confidentiality guidelines for participants in the nursing peer review process**

Peer Review Confidentiality Guidelines

The nursing review committee functions in accordance with the requirements of the (State) Nurse Practice Act. That article provides persons participating in good faith in the peer review process with extensive protection against incurring civil liability because of their participation. Without such protection, it would be very difficult for peer review committees to operate. It is necessary to protect not only the nurse being reviewed, but also to facilitate the open discussion of opinions by members and other participants in the process.

Violating these confidentiality provisions could result in exposure to civil liability both for the person breaching confidentiality and the committee itself.

The following guidelines are designed to assist participants to avoid any inadvertent breaches of confidentiality.

Restrictions on disclosure

1. A nursing peer review committee proceeding is **confidential**, and any communication made to the nursing peer review committee is privileged.
2. A member, agent, or employee may not disclose or be required to disclose any communication made to the committee or a record or proceeding of the committee.
3. A person who attends nursing peer review committee proceedings may not disclose or be required to disclose:
   a. Information acquired in connection with the proceedings
   b. An opinion, recommendation, or evaluation of the committee or a committee member
4. Members of the committee and participants may not be questioned about their testimony or about opinions formed as a result of the committee proceedings.
5. Peer review committee members are required to protect to the extent possible the identity of patients.

Recommendations

1. Do not discuss any case except as part of your official responsibilities on the committee. Casual or "cocktail" conversation about a case is one of the easiest ways to breach confidentiality. Discussing a case with a third party or expert to get his or her opinion

FIGURE 4.5 | **Confidentiality guidelines for participants in the nursing peer review process (cont'd.)**

or feeling can also result in inadvertently disclosing confidential information. You never know when some seemingly unimportant information will permit the third party to identify whom you are talking about.

2. If you are questioned about a case or your participation in a proceeding, you should respond that (name of your hospital) does not permit you to respond to any questions. Also, immediately notify the vice president of nursing or the vice president of quality.
3. Refer to individual patients by their medical record number only.
4. If you have any questions about confidentiality, consult the committee chair.

I have read the above guidelines and understand and agree to abide by them.

____________________________________ __________________

Name (Print) Date

____

Signature

Chapter 5

STEP 2

Establish the Nursing Peer Review Process

Learning objectives

After reading this chapter, the participant will be able to:

- Describe the case review process relating to committee review
- Identify referral sources for case reviews
- Identify when a case would need further review by a clinical expert
- List the process steps to take when care is deemed "appropriate" and "inappropriate"

Once an organization has made the decision to implement peer review and determined the structure, it is time to actually begin establishing the peer review process. It is crucial that the process have a systematic design and protected approach. This means creating a formal policy, charter, and process that you will follow as you perform nursing peer review. Doing so ensures that the program has the authority and validity it needs to be accepted and valued, as well as the system to ensure it runs smoothly.

Peer Review Policy

Hospitals are required by The Joint Commission to have a policy that defines the peer review process for the medical staff, and nursing peer review should follow this model. If your organization currently has a medical staff peer review process and policy in place, consider modeling the nursing peer review process on the medical staff's process.

The peer review process is protected under the federal Health Care Quality Improvement Act, as well as under any state statutes. Follow state statutes regarding peer review protection so you understand what is discoverable and how to protect the information.

Modeling the nursing peer review function on the medical staff peer review process is a first step toward establishing nursing peer review under the same protection.

Drafting a peer review policy

Start by creating a peer review policy, as it is the overriding document of the peer review process, laying it out in general strokes and guiding your organization throughout the process of fleshing it out.

The policy should have attachments that further define the process, including the peer review committee charter (included in Chapter 4 as Figure 4.4), a document setting forth the peer review process and timelines (which will be discussed in this chapter), a case review rating form (included in Chapter 7 as Figure 7.1), and a current list of nursing performance indicators and targets (see Chapter 8 for more details on performance indicators and targets).

The first step, the peer review policy, can be created new, adapted from the medical staff's policy, or based on the sample peer review policy shown in Figure 5.1. The policy outlines the scope, goals, and format of the peer review function. The members of the nursing peer review committee you establish should review your policy annually to check for any potential additions, deletions, or revisions that need to be made.

In addition to the policy, organizations should draft a document that outlines the steps in the process. The process and timelines document works in parallel with the policy and charter documents (see Chapter 4 for a copy of the charter).

FIGURE 5.1 | **Sample nursing peer review committee policy**

Nursing Peer Review Committee Policy

Purpose

To ensure that the hospital, through the activities of its nursing staff, assesses the performance of individuals (employee or contractor) and uses the results of such assessments to improve care.

Goals

1. Improve the quality of care provided by individual nurses
2. Monitor nurses' performance
3. Identify opportunities for performance improvement
4. Identify system process issues
5. Monitor significant trends by analyzing aggregate data
6. Ensure that the process for peer review is clearly defined, fair, defensible, timely, and useful

Definitions

Peer review

Peer review is the evaluation of an individual nurse's professional performance and includes the identification of opportunities to improve care.

Peer review differs from other quality improvement processes in that it evaluates the strengths and weaknesses of an individual nurse's performance, rather than appraising the quality of care rendered by a group of professionals or a system.

Peer review is conducted using multiple sources of information, including:

1. The review of individual cases
2. The review of aggregate data for compliance with general rules of the nursing staff
3. Clinical standards and use of rates in comparison with established benchmarks or norms

The individual's evaluation is based on generally recognized standards of care. Through this process, nurses receive feedback for personal improvement or confirmation of personal achievement related to the effectiveness of their professional, technical, and interpersonal skills in providing patient care. For specialty-specific clinical issues, such as evaluating the technique of a specialized procedure, a peer is an individual who is well trained and competent in that specialty.

FIGURE 5.1 **Sample nursing peer review committee policy (cont'd.)**

The degree of subject matter expertise required for a provider to be considered a peer for all peer reviews performed by or on behalf of the hospital will be determined by the nursing peer review committee (NPRC) unless otherwise designated for specific circumstances by nursing leadership.

Conflict of interest

A conflict of interest exists if a member of the nursing staff is not able to render an unbiased opinion. Automatic conflict of interests would result if the nurse on the peer review committee is the nurse under review. Relative conflicts of interest are due to the reviewer either being involved in the patient's care or having a familial relationship with the nurse involved, and similar situations.

It is the obligation of the individual reviewer to disclose to the peer review committee the potential conflict. The responsibility of the peer review body is to determine whether the conflict would prevent the individual from participating or the extent of the individual's participation. Individuals determined to have a conflict may not be present during peer review body discussions or decisions other than to provide information if requested.

Policy

1. All peer review information is privileged and confidential in accordance with nursing and hospital bylaws, state and federal laws, and regulations pertaining to confidentiality and nondiscoverability.
2. The involved nurse will receive specific feedback on a case-by-case basis.
3. The hospital will use the nurse-specific peer review results in its annual evaluation process, and as appropriate, in its performance improvement activities.
4. The hospital will keep nurse-specific peer review and other quality information concerning a nurse in a secure, locked file archived in nursing administration. The peer review and quality information will be kept separate from the employment file. Nurse-specific peer review information consists of information related to:
    - Performance data for all dimensions of performance measured for that individual nurse
    - The individual nurse's role in sentinel events, significant incidents, or near misses
    - Correspondence to the nurse regarding commendations, comments regarding practice performance, or corrective action

FIGURE 5.1 **Sample nursing peer review committee policy (cont'd.)**

5. Peer review information is available only to authorized individuals who have a legitimate need to know this information based upon their responsibilities as a nursing leader or hospital employee. However, they shall have access to the information only to the extent necessary to carry out their assigned responsibilities. Only the following individuals shall have access to nurse-specific peer review information and only for purposes of quality improvement:
   - Vice president, nursing
   - Administrative director, nursing operations
   - Individuals surveying for accrediting bodies with appropriate jurisdiction (e.g., The Joint Commission or state/federal regulatory bodies)
   - Individuals with a legitimate purpose for access as determined by the hospital board of directors
6. No copies of peer review documents will be created and distributed unless authorized by the vice president of nursing, or per hospital policy.

Circumstances requiring peer review

Peer review is conducted on an ongoing basis and reported to the NPRC for review and action. The procedure for conducting peer review is described in the "Process and time frames" document. Evaluation of a case will be conducted through the following means:

- Through reporting processes such as occurrence reports
- When there is a sentinel event or "near miss" identified during concurrent or retrospective review
- When there is an unusual individual case or clinical pattern of care identified during a quality review

Circumstances requiring external peer review

The NPRC will make recommendations on the need for external peer review to nursing leadership. External peer review will take place under the following circumstances if deemed appropriate by nursing leadership or by the board of directors.

FIGURE 5.1 **Sample nursing peer review committee policy (cont'd.)**

A nurse cannot require the hospital to obtain external peer review if it is not deemed appropriate by the nursing leadership or board of directors.

Circumstances requiring external peer review include:

- Litigation—when dealing with the potential for a lawsuit.
- Ambiguity—when dealing with vague or conflicting recommendations from internal reviewers and conclusions from this review will directly affect a nurse's employment.
- Lack of internal expertise—when no one on the nursing staff has adequate expertise in the specialty under review, or when the only nurse with that expertise is determined to have a conflict of interest regarding the nurse under review as described above. External peer review will take place if this potential for conflict of interest cannot be appropriately resolved by nursing leadership.
- Miscellaneous issues—when the nursing staff needs an expert for purposes of establishing nursing standards.

Participants in the review process

Participants in the review process will be selected according to the nursing policies and procedures. Medical staff will participate in the review process if deemed appropriate.

Additional support staff will participate if such participation is included in their job responsibilities.

The NPRC will consider and record the views of the person whose care is under review prior to making a final determination regarding the care provided by that individual, as long as the individual responds in the time frame outlined.

In the event of a conflict of interest or circumstances that would suggest a biased review, the NPRC and nursing leadership will determine who will participate in the process.

Participants with a conflict of interest may not be present.

FIGURE 5.1 **Sample nursing peer review committee policy (cont'd.)**

Thresholds for intensive review

If the results of individual case reviews for a nurse exceed thresholds established by the nursing staff (described below), the NPRC will review the findings to determine whether further intensive review is needed to identify a potential pattern of care.

Thresholds:

- Any single egregious case
- Within any 12-month period of time, any one of the following criteria:
  - Three cases rated "care inappropriate"
  - Five cases rated either care controversial or inappropriate
  - Five cases rated as having documentation issues regardless of care rating

Peer review for specific circumstances

In the event a decision is made by the board of directors to investigate a nurse's performance or circumstances warrant the evaluation of one or more providers, the professional practice chair council or its designee shall appoint a panel of appropriate nursing professionals to perform the necessary peer review activities.

Peer review time frames

Peer review will be conducted by the peer review committee in a timely manner. The goal is for routine cases to be completed within 90 days from the date the chart is reviewed by the QM coordinator and complex cases to be completed within 120 days. Exceptions may occur based on case complexity or reviewer availability.

Statutory authority

The above policy is based on the statutory authority of the Health Care Quality Improvement Act of 1986 42 U.S.C. 11101, et seq. and State law: ____ (Insert your state's law here).

Peer Review Process and Timelines

An effective committee structure must outline each one of the steps of the peer review system, starting with the point of referral and how referrals are made to the committee, and ending with the final step, which is the final committee determination.

The elapsed time between cases occurring and being referred to the committee will differ on a case-by-case basis. Serious incidents will likely be referred immediately, whereas less severe incidents may take a little longer to be referred. This potential lag time needs to be discussed when educating staff about the new peer review process. All staff members need to be aware of how and why cases should be referred to the peer review committee, both to ensure that appropriate cases are referred and that they are referred in a timely manner.

Charts may be referred to nursing peer review by a variety of sources, though most often by referrals, coders, or quality or risk personnel.

Cases may be referred by any of the following:

- Nursing leadership
- Hospital departments or employees
- Medical staff members and members of the medical staff peer review committee
- Risk management
- Patient representatives
- Payers
- State organizations
- General screens

Once cases have been identified as potentially requiring review, begin the process with the goal that these cases move through the case review process in 90 days or less, with the understanding that some cases may extend longer due to the severity of the case or because the case raises additional questions that need to be addressed either by the nurse involved or by other parties.

The timeline of the entire process of identifying, scoring, and then determining the outcome of the case is outlined in Figure 5.2, the process and timelines document, and will be discussed in the rest of the chapter. Figure 5.3 provides a flowchart example of the process.

FIGURE 5.2 **Nursing peer review process and time frames**

Topic	Case review process	Timeline guidelines
Case identification	Charts identified by HIM coders, quality/risk personnel. Patient case review work list screened for indicators by the quality database system. Cases identified by incident reports with adequate information for review available.	Quality management (QM) coordinator informed about the chart when the chart is complete or within 30 days of patient discharge, whichever occurs first. Charts requested from work lists by quality analyst within two weeks of discharge. Identified cases sent to the QM coordinator within two days of case identification.
Case screening	Quality analyst reviews cases to determine whether they are acceptable. If nurse review is required, the chart is assigned to nurse reviewer per the nursing peer review committee (NPRC) policy. The quality analyst provides the reviewer a case summary and identifies key issues.	Quality analyst will perform the initial screen and assign the case to nurse reviewer within one week of receiving the chart.
Nurse review	Nurse reviewer reviews case and completes review section of Nursing Peer Review Form.	Review will be completed within two weeks of assigning chart.
Additional review needed	If additional expertise is required (either internal or external), initial reviewer will contact the nursing peer review chair or designee to determine second reviewer, unless the second reviewer is a nursing peer review member.	Second review to be completed within two weeks of assigning chart unless difficulty is encountered obtaining second reviewer.

FIGURE 5.2 | **Nursing peer review process and time frames (cont'd.)**

Topic	Case review process	Timeline guidelines
Completed case review	Completed reviews will be submitted to the quality analyst by the nurse reviewer immediately to enter into the case review tracking system.	Completed reviews must be submitted to the quality analyst three days prior to the NPRC meeting to be included in the agenda.
Reviews rated care appropriate	Reviews indicating appropriate nursing care are reported to the NPRC for summary approval.	Appropriate care reviews are approved at the next meeting after the review is submitted.
Reviews rated questionable or care inappropriate	Reviews indicating controversial or inappropriate nursing care are presented to the NPRC for discussion and confirmation or change in preliminary scoring. If the committee feels that care may be controversial or inappropriate, it will communicate with the involved nurse(s) by letter. The involved nurse(s) are informed of the key questions regarding the case and asked to respond. If care is determined to be appropriate, the nurse will be informed as described below.	Nurse under review will respond to committee within two weeks. If no response, the nurse will be notified by letter to respond within two weeks, or the committee will finalize rating based on the available information. The nursing office will contact the nurse by phone to determine whether the nurse is unavailable due to special circumstances.
Communicating findings to nurses	For cases determined as **appropriate** nursing care, involved nurses are informed of the decision by routine letter. For cases of **inappropriate** or **controversial** care, involved nurses are informed of the decision by nursing leadership and a copy of the letter will be archived in the nursing peer review file.	Appropriate care letters sent to nurse(s) under review within 30 days of the NPRC meeting.

FIGURE 5.2 | **Nursing peer review process and time frames (cont'd.)**

Improvement plan process		
Improvement plan development	If the results of either case reviews or analysis of rate or rule indicator trends indicate a need for individual nurse performance improvement, the issue will be referred to the appropriate nursing director/manager. The NPRC chair and the nursing director/manager will work together to create and implement the improvement action plan.	The nursing director/manager and the NPRC chair will create and implement the improvement plan within 30 days. The QM department will track the improvement implementation and the date implemented and will report back to the NPRC.
Referrals to hospital committees	For cases with potential opportunities for improving system performance or potential issues with nursing care, the NPRC will communicate the issue to the appropriate hospital committee.	The hospital committee receiving the referral will discuss the issue and communicate the action plan to the referring committee.

High-risk case timelines

For high-risk cases, timely processing of nurse-specific information is necessary to ensure patient safety. For sentinel events requiring peer review, immediate review by the NPRC chair or designee will be performed within 72 hours of identification, with committee action/decision within 45 days of the event.

Additional information (e.g., literature searches, second opinion, or external peer review) may be necessary before making a decision or action. Under these circumstances, the timelines may be extended after approval from the governing body or its designee.

The case review process proceeds in the following fundamental manner:

1. Case identification
2. Case screening and assigning of nurse reviewer
3. Nurse review
4. Additional review
5. Completed case review
6. Reviewers rate cases as "care appropriate," and the process ceases
7. Reviewers rate cases as "questionable or inappropriate care," and the process continues
8. An inquiry letter is sent to the nurse involved asking for his or her input on the case
9. Communication of findings to nurses
10. Tracking review findings

The process flow chart shown in Figure 5.3 reflects the step-by-step algorithm for case review. The chart is useful when working with the peer review committee members to assist them in understanding the decisions and process to follow after selection of a case.

FIGURE 5.3 **Process flow chart**

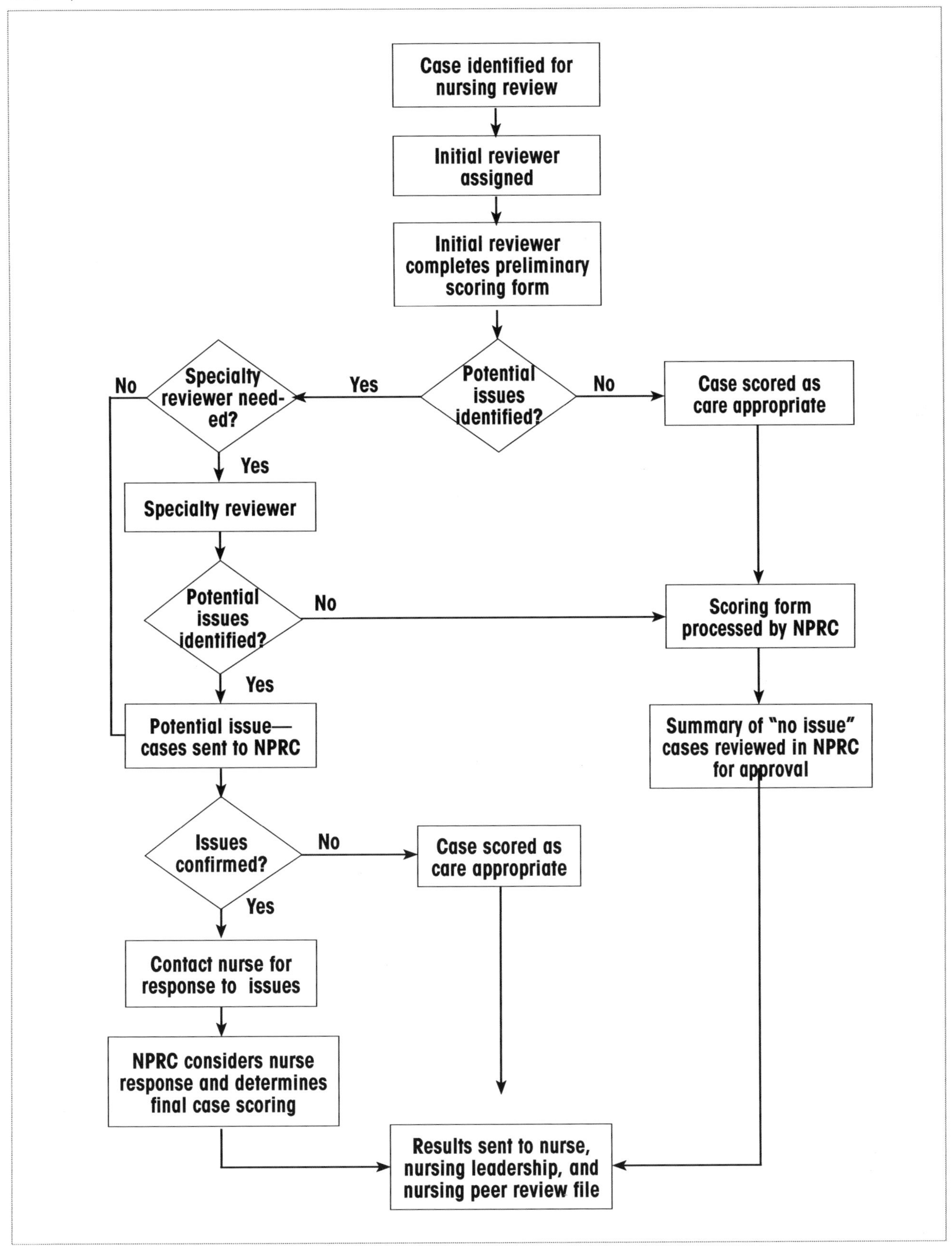

Case identification

When cases are referred for potential review by the nursing peer review committee, there must be a defined list of screening criteria and indicators established to identify those referrals that will be accepted for review by the nurse reviewers and the nursing peer review committee. Basically, the screening criteria and indicators are nursing quality indicators chosen for review because there is determined high risk or a problem for the organization.

Performance measures, also called indicators, do more than provide data—they indicate how something is actually performing. These criteria are outlined in Chapter 8, where review indicators are discussed in detail.

Case screening and assignment of nurse reviewer

Referrals need to be handled by one person who knows the criteria for cases selected for peer review. This person is the quality analyst or screener and performs an important gatekeeper role, so care should be taken in assigning a person to this role. If your organization does not have a quality analyst or screener, then the chair of the peer review committee can perform this role.

The quality analyst or screener may be a nurse or an analyst from the quality department. It is important that the person in this role has a high comfort level with the committee and with the criteria for what is suitable for peer review, and, as such, it is often useful if the person possesses clinical experience.

Once the members of the peer review committee decide who the quality analyst will be, this person becomes a member of the committee but does not have voting rights in the final committee decisions.

When a case is brought to the quality analyst, it should take no more than one week before it is determined whether it will be submitted for nurse review. The quality analyst creates a case summary, identifies key issues, and presents this information in a packet that will be submitted to the nurse reviewer for initial screening. Some committees may assign the quality analyst position an administrative role and have this person responsible for assembling all packets for full committee review and for taking minutes during meetings.

The quality analyst uses the decided-upon indicators as criteria for sending a case to nurse review, but if the person is ever unsure about whether a case meets criteria, it should be submitted to nurse review anyway.

Determining who will perform this key position is crucial. Some of the key responsibilities and roles of the quality analyst are listed in Figure 5.4.

FIGURE 5.4 **Job summary and skills inventory for quality analyst/screener role**

Technical skills	• Performs routine and intensive medical record audits based on submitted referrals for peer review • Ensures compliance with applicable regulatory guidelines and requirements; state and federal statutes; and nursing peer review bylaws, rules, and policies • Coordinates outside reviews when requested by the nursing staff • Maintains all electronic/hard-copy documentation of case review outcomes • Provides the nursing peer review committee with committee-based performance summaries • Is able to plan and effectively organize work
Service focus	• Supports peer review committee functions and the flow of information to nursing staff groups and hospital departments • Develops positive working relationships with the nursing staff through responsiveness and delivery of accurate, timely, and effective work products • Assists with and supports nursing staff education regarding peer review and regulatory requirements
Job knowledge	• Remains current with peer review state statutes and federal requirements • Is able to understand and apply information, policies, procedures, and skills required by the position • Is computer proficient with applicable hardware and software • Collaborates effectively, efficiently, and appropriately with nursing leadership and nursing staff
Communications	• Expresses thoughts clearly and concisely (verbal and written) • Formulates all peer review case feedback letters from the committee to nurses involved in specific cases • Formulates all peer review committee meeting agendas and case packets, and captures meeting minutes • Keeps all necessary people informed and up to date • Projects poise and credibility in meetings • Maintains the confidentiality of all business/work and nursing staff information
Supervision required	• Independently carries out instructions and responsibilities and follows through with affected parties/areas • Seeks assistance appropriately • Uses resources in an appropriate and cost-effective manner

This initial review helps ensure that the issues of the case are nursing related. After the initial review, the quality analyst gives the case summary and any key questions to the nurse reviewer. Cases are assigned to reviewers on a rotating basis or may be based on specialty-specific expertise.

Evaluation by the nurse reviewer

Identifying charts for potential review is the first step in the process, but the real investigation of the issues and concerns begins when the nurse reviewer looks at the case and chart. The process of how to conduct a review is covered in depth in Chapter 7, but it is important to consider what kind of scoring your organization will use at this point, so that you can establish the timeline for the rest of the process.

For cases to be reviewed effectively and efficiently, there must be a standardized method of evaluating cases so that each reviewer looks at cases in the same way. If committees are to reach consensus, they must use some form of standardized scoring.

Once the case has been assigned to a nurse on the peer review committee, the nurse reviewer should be given two weeks to complete his or her review. The completed case review form should then promptly be given back to the quality analyst/screener. The case review form should be returned to the quality analyst at least three days prior to a scheduled committee meeting so that there is time for the case to be placed on the agenda.

If the nurse reviewer is uncertain about the case and how to score it, he or she has two options: Either the case may be reassigned to a different nurse reviewer on the committee prior to a committee meeting, or the reviewer can discuss the case and his or her thoughts and concerns in the committee forum.

If the nurse reviewer lacks the expertise to make a determination on the case, then the appropriate clinical nursing expert needs to be obtained prior to the committee meeting.

If the nurse reviewer deems the overall case as "appropriate," then the case does not proceed any further in the peer review process. The nurse involved in the case being reviewed should be informed of the review outcome by letter. (Sample letter templates can be found in Chapter 7.)

If the nurse reviewer finds the case to be "controversial" or "inappropriate," then it is placed on the committee meeting agenda to be discussed by all members of the peer review committee. During the committee meeting, all members will discuss the basis for the reviewer's findings and will outline any questions pertaining to the case review.

Additional review as needed

After the initial review by the nurse reviewer, you may have cause to conduct an additional review. This may occur if the case involved more than one issue and/or more than one nurse, or if the nurse reviewer feels that the case issues presented in the review are outside of his or her specialty or knowledge. The nurse reviewer will need to notify the quality analyst/screener or the chair of the committee so the case can be reassigned to the appropriate clinical expert(s).

If a case involves multiple nurses, then each nurse should be treated individually and his or her actions evaluated separately, because there may be entirely different issues to be examined for individual nurses, even if it involves the same patient situation or outcome.

Completed case review

Once the nurse reviewer has reviewed the case, he or she must promptly return the case form to the quality analyst/screener to be placed on the next month's agenda for the committee. The nurse reviewer must give the quality analyst enough time to prepare packets to distribute to the full committee during the meeting.

If the nurse reviewer does not submit the case form to the quality analyst within three days prior to the meeting, the case should be deferred to the following month's committee meeting.

Reviews rated as care appropriate

The nurse reviewer may determine that the care provided in the case is satisfactory and confer a "care appropriate" rating on the situation. That case is then aggregated by the quality analyst and entered into the peer review records. The committee chair will meet with the quality analyst prior to the meeting to review all care appropriate cases to sign off or determine if a discussion is needed on specific cases during the time of the meeting. All other care appropriate determinations will be discussed briefly as a summary.

The nurse involved in the case is also sent a letter informing him or her that the case has been deemed as having "no issue" or as "care appropriate" and no further action is necessary.

Reviews rated as questionable or inappropriate care

If the nurse reviewer feels the case is either care controversial or care inappropriate, the case will be placed on the agenda for the next meeting, and the committee members will discuss the case within the group.

During the committee meeting, the initial nurse reviewer will discuss the case and how he or she came to the initial scoring, and the nurse reviewer will present to the group the key questions that have been generated regarding the involved nurse.

It is important to note that the initial review of the case needs to happen prior to the scheduled committee meeting date. Reviews should not be done at the time of the meeting.

The nurse or nurses involved in a case should be given an option to respond to the committee and clarify any questions or issues that have been raised. When the committee deems a case to be care controversial or care inappropriate, questions will be generated that can be sent to the nurse in a letter. This gives the involved nurse the opportunity to respond to the questions generated by committee review prior to the committee making its final determination on a case.

The involved nurse should be given two weeks to respond to the committee's questions. If the nurse fails to respond, a second inquiry letter should be sent extending the time period an additional two weeks. If a response is still not received, the committee should make a determination without the nurse's input.

If the nurse does respond to the inquiry letter, it should be done in writing. If the involved nurse needs further clarification about the questions being asked, he or she should inquire through his or her nurse managers and then discuss this with the committee chairperson.

Communicating findings to nurses

After receiving the nurse's response, the committee discusses the case and finalizes the ratings. The committee will then notify the nurse of the final determination by a letter sent via certified mail. The committee may decide to give a copy of the letter to the nurse manager or supervisor who oversees the nurse's patient care.

The committee will also send letters to nurses to identify any potential exemplary care or exemplary documentation that was found during the course of the review.

Recognition: Accentuate the positive!

Be sure to recognize staff who meet the nursing expectations, and set aside time to celebrate exceptional performance.

Recognizing outstanding performance improves the nursing culture—it creates a positive environment which will result in improved outcomes. Your nurses will recognize that your peer review process truly is nonpunitive.

Tracking review findings

Cases examined by the peer review committee need to be tracked and trended. The organization should determine the best way to track the findings of the case review process.

Ideally, the committee will track cases electronically, and organizations may want to use a software program purchased from an outside vendor or create their own spreadsheets to track cases. Tracking cases electronically will also offer a more confidential and secure process.

Chapter 6

STEP 3

Educate Nurse and Nonnurse Stakeholders

Learning objectives

After reading this chapter, the participant will be able to:

- Relate the importance of educating nurses and nonnurse stakeholders on the peer review process
- Identify communication methods that are effective during the implementation process
- List ways to reduce fear among nurses regarding the peer review process

The final step to complete before you can schedule a committee meeting to review your organization's first case is to ensure that everyone understands the goals and intentions of the new peer review process. One of the dangers in implementing a new program is that if nurses do not understand the process, they may mistakenly believe that it is a disciplinary council and that its purpose is to punish nurses if they make a mistake.

Communicating the Mission

Before the program is up and running, you must make it clear to nurses that peer review is about improving the quality of care they provide and is dedicated to patient safety. They also need to know that the process is about *nurses discussing nursing care* and that it is nonpunitive. And the education should not stop at nurses—it is vital that others in the organization understand the process as well.

Targeting the audience

Educating staff members about the new peer review process should occur during the design phase and prior to the committee's first review meeting. As you can imagine, educating stakeholders (nurses), union representatives, nonstakeholders (e.g., risk and quality managers), and committee members is an essential and a critical part of the design process. If it is not done properly, nurses become guarded and may assume that the new process is for punitive reasons.

It is crucial to begin the education process as soon as possible, and it is imperative that it be done before an actual review is conducted. It would not be pleasant for a nurse to receive a letter from the nursing peer review committee or inquiries regarding a case review if he or she was not aware of the new process.

Therefore, after creating the structure to support nursing peer review, when you are ready for implementation, the next step is to educate the nurses and nonstakeholders prior to implementation.

The target audience who needs education includes:

- Nursing staff
- Union representatives
- Hospital and medical staff leadership
- Quality and risk management professionals
- Board of directors/trustees

In most organizations, there are different forums you can use to communicate with and educate all staff, and a successful program implementation should make use of many of these. Part of the planning process should involve developing a communication plan that will meet the needs of your organization. This plan should include a variety of methods of communication to ensure that there are multiple ways to communicate with nurses and other staff. As you can imagine, communicating with the different shifts of nurses might be different and needs to be part of the plan.

Your organization may have various standing committees or meetings that provide ready-made opportunities for discussion, in which case you can create a formal presentation explaining the process and present it during these meetings. This type of communication is beneficial because it gives the staff time to ask the questions that are worrying them.

Other options include creating newsletters or brochures that nurses can read on their own time. Also make use of all technological opportunities you have, including flat-screen communication boards, email bulletins, your organization's intranet, or the facility's Web page.

Do not use one method and assume everyone is on board. When communicating the new program to staff, make sure to include a variety of methods across an extended period of time to ensure that everyone has heard your message. Use as many as necessary from the effective communication tools in this list:

- Committees or other meetings
- Nursing educational software
- Flat-screen communication boards
- Email bulletins or updates
- Staff newsletters
- Internet sites
- Intranet bulletin boards
- Memorandums included in/with paychecks
- Posters and bulletins boards
- Flyers and brochures

Designate a day for training

One of the best ways to provide initial education to a large number of people, and thus attempt to reach all the people who need to be informed, is to hold an educational training session. This gives you a captive audience so you can thoroughly explain the components of peer review and allow time for discussion and questions.

Some organizations may designate a day as the "peer review kickoff" and schedule duplicate one-hour meetings throughout the day. This allows you to stagger the number of patient care nurses attending the meeting and decrease the amount of staff leaving one unit at any one time.

This is an effective way to communicate to the target audience, and it provides an excellent forum for interactive discussion. Make this meeting mandatory so that all nurses participate and follow up the meeting with unit meetings, newsletter articles, and posters to reinforce the goals and objectives of the new process.

NOTE > Make sure that your peer review discussion is added to the orientation process so that all new nurses joining the organization understand what is expected of them from the first day on the job.

Also, make sure peer review discussion is added to the orientation process so that all new nurses joining the organization understand what is expected of them from the first day on the job.

It is imperative that throughout all the educational outreaches, whether through newsletter articles or formal presentations, the patient care aspect is stressed, but also state that although the new process does look at issues related to patient care, it also acknowledges excellence in care and documentation.

Involving nonnurse stakeholders

The focus of the peer review process is on nursing care and overall nurse performance, but we also want to involve any nonnursing stakeholders, such as risk and quality managers, who will be among those referring cases to the committee so that they understand the process for referring a case to the committee.

In addition, it is helpful to ensure that medical staff representatives are involved in the education phases, because in the event that the nursing peer review process identifies a physician component or medical quality concern, the issue will be forwarded to the appropriate medical staff committee for review.

Eliminating fear and obtaining buy-in

Adding a new committee to the current nursing structure will always provoke some questioning from staff, and many will question the intent of the committee. This is why it is crucial to reinforce that this is not a punitive process and to ensure staff that although nursing peer review does provide information regarding nursing performance, the real goals of implementing this process are to:

- Improve the quality of care provided by individual nurses
- Monitor the performance of nurses
- Identify opportunities for performance improvement
- Identify systemwide issues

While discussing peer review, let nurses know that some case reviews identify system failure issues that cause human error, and others may identify situations in which it is simply a human error (e.g., giving 10 times the prescribed dose of insulin to a patient even though the medication is labeled accurately).

Let them know that even without the peer review process, some level of action is always taken to educate the nurse to prevent future errors. The difference now is that the formal review process provides a mechanism for "peers" to review the episode and make a determination without nursing leadership.

> **NOTE >** You cannot stress this often enough: Peer review enables nurses to take responsibility for their own profession.

Other ways to eliminate fear through education are to:

- Provide a sample case scoring form, information about the case review process, and other pertinent documents to the nurses during the education session
- Provide the PowerPoint slides for any presentations in handout materials so nurses may review them later
- Identify committee members
- Ensure that the chief nursing officer is present during the educational sessions to reinforce the nonpunitive process
- Provide ongoing communication and updates to take the "unknown" out of the equation

Conducting a formal presentation

Formal presentations are one of the easiest ways to educate large groups of people about the new process. The following sample PowerPoint presentation will walk you through how to explain the process to staff nurses, nonnurse stakeholders, and committee members to reduce their fears. You can easily modify the presentation for the selected audience and to appeal to target groups.

The text following the PowerPoint slides highlights the crucial aspects to pull out during your presentation, as well as some additional information you may wish to include. The presentation is included with the downloadable resources—use it as is or adapt for your own needs. Find the PowerPoint at *www.hcpro.com/downloads/12285*.

CONTEMPORARY APPROACHES
for Implementing
Nursing Peer Review

Who "owns" quality of care at your healthcare organization?

Answer:

Ultimately, the Board...

But each licensed professional is responsible for his or her own individual actions

The board of directors/trustees is ultimately held accountable for the quality of care provided in your organization.

Why do we do peer review?

The bottom line:

Nurses are mutually accountable to each other for the quality of care they provide

Note that physicians have been holding each other accountable for decades; nurses should have the same standards and evaluate their care.

What is nursing peer review?

What does The Joint Commission want?

- *For the process to be consistent, timely, defensible, balanced, and useful*

What are we really trying to do?

- *Evaluate and improve nursing performance*

Is chart review the only way to evaluate performance?

- *Chart review is one of the most useful components to evaluate patient care and to encourage nurses to be accountable for their profession*

Chart review is not the only way to evaluate performance, and the organization will use other methods. However, chart review is one of the most useful components to evaluate patient care and to encourage nurses to be accountable for their profession.

Examples of peer review might be an OB nurse reviewing the case of another OB nurse or a medical-surgical nurse reviewing the case of a medical-surgical nurse.

It can be worth offering a brief overview of the different types of peer review, but this discussion may be dependent on your audience. For example, you might want to omit this slide for audiences consisting of leadership, the quality committee, or the board of directors/trustees. Nurses would be most interested in this information.

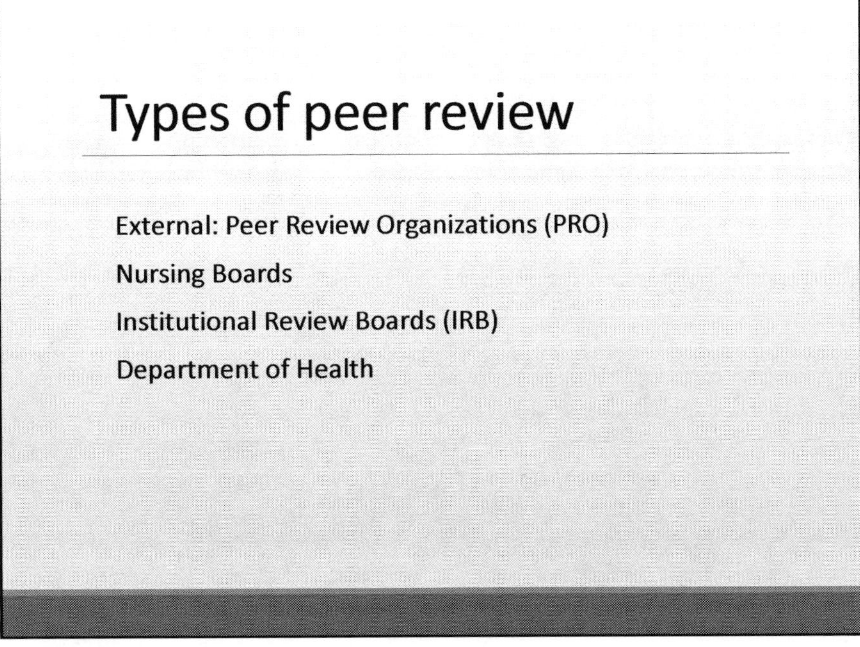

If you choose to include more details about the types of peer review, you can find more information in Chapter 1.

Note, however, that you should spend a considerable amount of time on the goals of peer review so that nurses understand why the new program is being initiated. Take a look at the following slides.

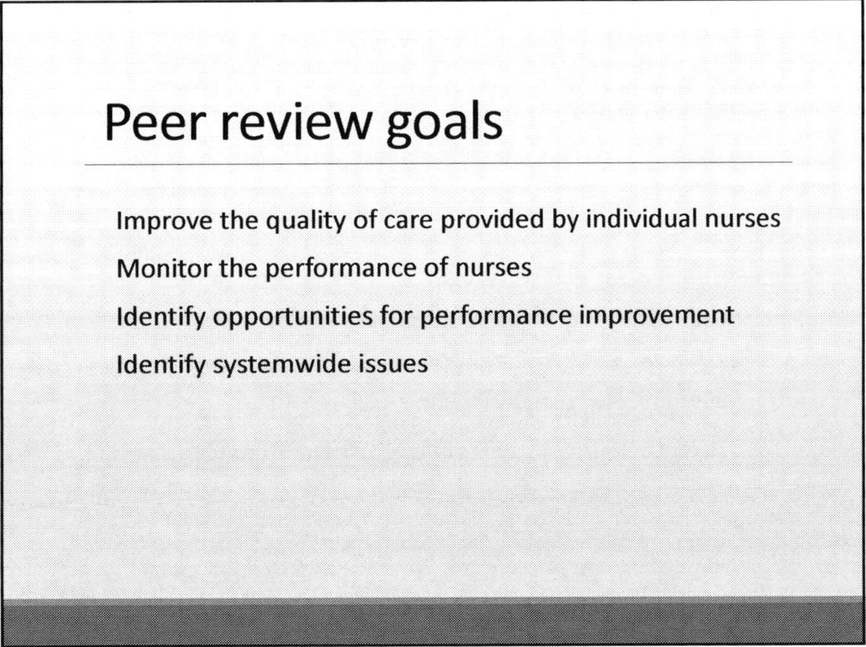

This is also the time to discuss expectations particular for your facility. Use the following nursing performance pyramid as an illustration.

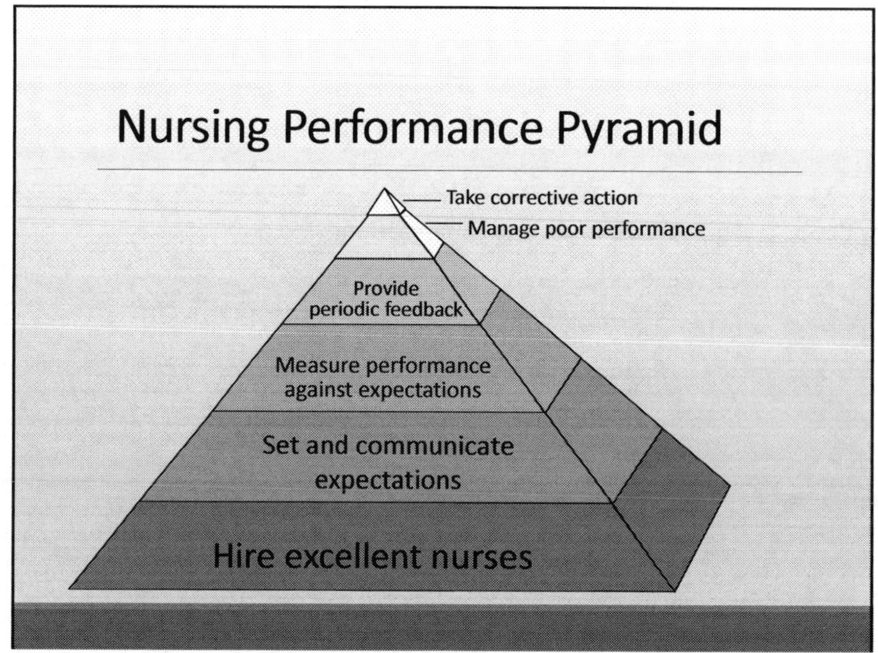

The nursing peer review process is part of the "measure performance against expectations" section of the pyramid. This is discussed in more detail in Chapter 2.

After presenting the pyramid, you can detail the six steps to implementing peer review that your organization has been working on. See the following nine slides for these points.

Six steps to achieve effective peer review

1. Define performance expectations
2. Link performance to expectations
3. Use all types of indicators
4. Standardize the review process
5. Create a nursing peer review structure
6. Provide effective feedback

STEP 1
Define performance expectations

- Technical
- Service
- Resource
- Relationships
- Citizenship

STEP 2
Link performance to expectations

How do we choose performance measures for annual evaluation?

- Job description
- Competency assessments
- 360-degree evaluation (coworker [peer] evaluation)
- Policies (e.g., code of conduct)
- Peer review

STEP 3
Use all types of indicators

Categorize all nursing indicators into three types:

- Type I: Rules
- Type II: Review
- Type III: Rates

Type 1: Rule-based indicators are related to nursing/hospital policy (e.g., nursing assessment not performed within 24 hours of admission).

Type 2: Review-based indicators require nurses to review the case to draw a conclusion regarding care. This involves case review, which is included in the peer review committee responsibilities.

Type 3: Rate-based indicators are typically represented as a percent of compliance (e.g., completion of nursing assessment within 24 hours of admission, flu and pneumonia vaccination documented, or documentation of smoking cessation information).

STEP 4
Standardize the case review process

- Clarify and communicate the basis for case selection
- Define the review focus to create a more efficient review process
- Design and implement an effective peer review scoring model
- Create and implement reviewer and staff expectations for the review procedure
- Decrease bias, increase fairness and defensibility
- Make performance feedback and training easy

STEP 5
Create a nursing peer review structure

- Informal vs. formal structure
- Use an existing committee, if possible, to centralize the peer review functions

This structure would be used for a shared governance model.

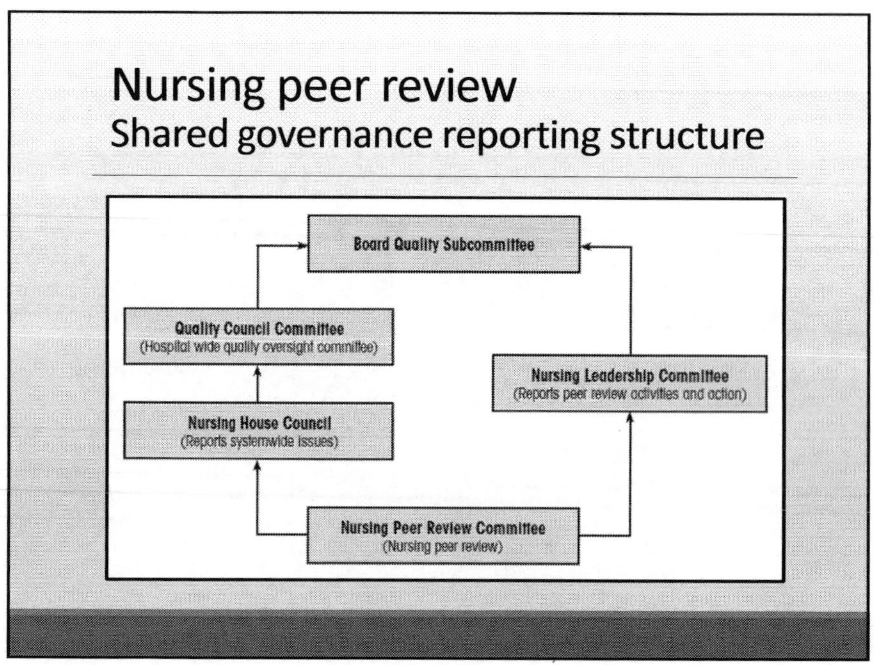

This structure would be used for all other types of nursing models.

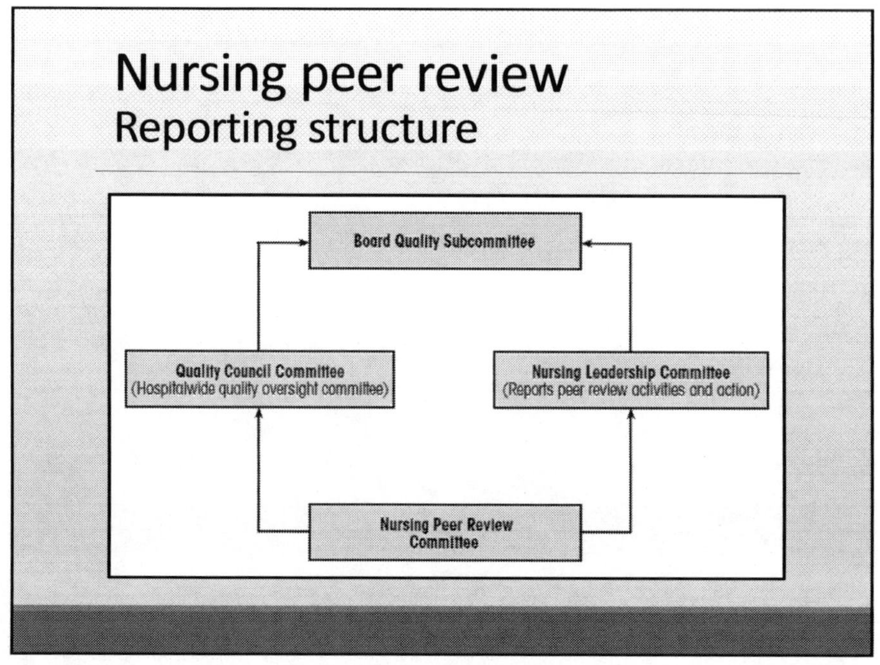

STEP 6
Provide effective feedback

1. Systematic and timely
2. Collegial and helpful
3. Positive and negative
4. Use data as a starting point for identifying improvement opportunities

Explain that cases should be reviewed as soon as possible after identification or referral. After a case has been through the process, explain that nursing can use the data to identify where potential areas of opportunity exist, which may lead to staff education as a whole on a new piece of equipment or on a process that has just been implemented.

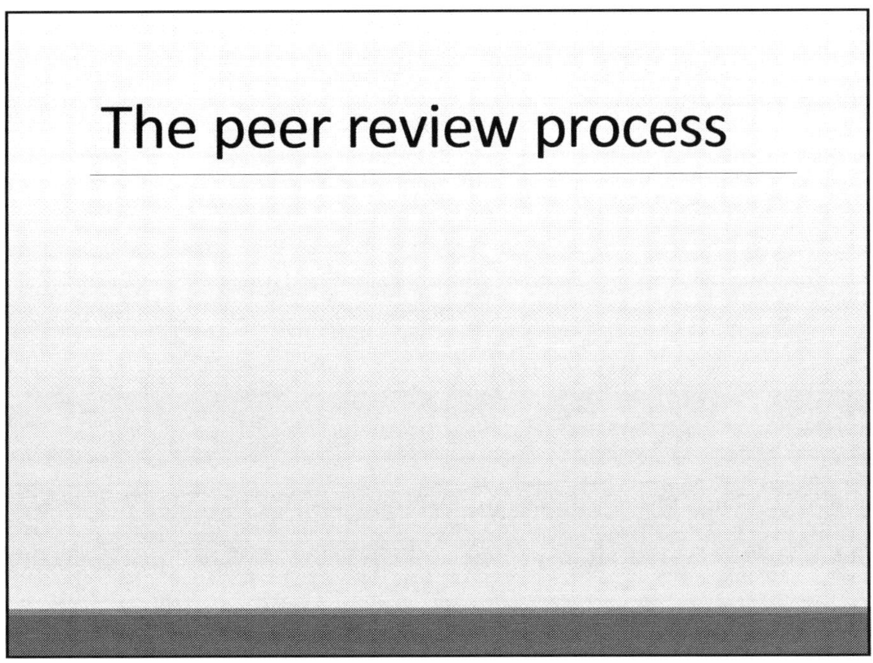

Purpose of the committee

In a nonpunitive manner, identify and communicate:

1. Nursing, department, unit, or systems issues
2. Issues deserving intense analysis
3. Educational opportunities

Case selection for review

- Quality of care (critical thinking)
- Technical errors
- Documentation
- Risk issues
- Complaints
- Other

Explain how cases are screened by a quality analyst and chair or designee prior to being forwarded to a committee member to ensure that any irrelevant cases are screened out. Offer examples of cases that are not appropriate for peer review, such as a disruptive outburst from a nurse, which would not be reviewed by the peer review committee because it is a discipline issue that should be addressed by the nurse's manager or nursing leadership.

How cases are referred

Cases may be referred by any of the following:

- Hospital departments or employees
- Medical staff members and members of the Medical Staff Peer Review Committee
- Risk management
- Patient representatives
- Patients
- Families
- Payers
- State organizations

Who reviews the charts

- Clinical experts (a clinical expert is a peer from the same discipline with essentially equal or similar qualifications)
- Ancillary departments may be contacted as needed for information

Explain that once a case is screened prior to the committee meeting, it may be necessary to obtain the review of a clinical expert who is not already represented on the committee to provide his or her clinical expertise during the case review. Invite the clinical expert to the committee, require a signed confidential statement, and then proceed with the case review.

How charts are reviewed

- Nurse reviewer (the clinical expert) reviews cases when notified
- Nurse reviewer recommends a determination or asks for more information from one or more referral sources, including the nurse involved

This slide is critical in your education of nurses, because being approached by the peer review committee members about a case can be a scary prospect for most nurses. Take time to explain that the peer review committee is simply trying to elicit as much information about a case as possible to come to a fair and balanced conclusion. It is in the nurse's best interests to be open and honest with the peer review committee. Explain that the nurse will not be punished by the committee; the peer review committee is simply trying to establish what happened so that lessons can be learned and systems improved.

If you receive a letter:

- Answer the questions to the best of your ability
- If you need help with the questions, feel free to contact the point person designated in the letter
- Respond to the letter within 14 days
- After the committee makes a decision, you will receive another letter with details

At this point, provide a copy of the blank case review form used by nurse reviewers to the nursing staff members in the audience. Understanding how charts are reviewed will help them feel more comfortable with the new process.

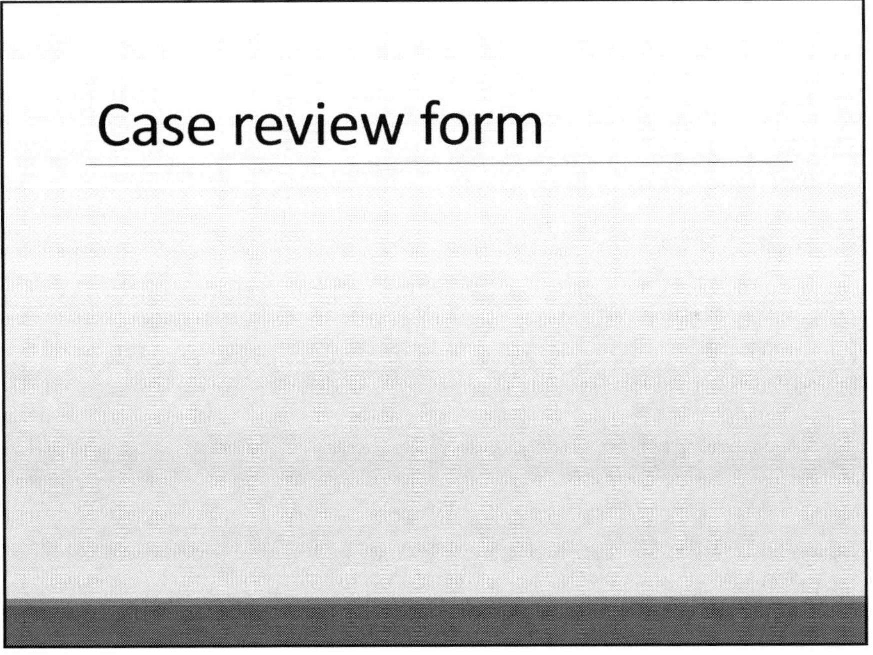

Then walk the audience through how the committee uses the form.

Use an effective
peer review scoring model

Basic categories to evaluate care:

- Patient outcome
- Effect on patient care
- Issue identification
- Documentation
- Overall nursing care (i.e., management)

Peer review scoring model: Outcomes

- No adverse outcome
- Minor adverse outcome (complete recovery expected)
- Major adverse outcome (complete recovery NOT expected)
- Catastrophic adverse outcome (e.g., death)

Peer review scoring model: Documentation

- No documentation issues
- Documentation does not substantiate clinical course and treatment
- Documentation not timely to communicate with other caregivers
- Documentation unreadable

Peer review scoring model: Issue identification

- Clinical thinking
- Assessment
- Technique/skills
- Knowledge
- Communication
- Planning
- Follow-up/follow-through
- Policy compliance
- Supervision (student)
- Other

Peer review scoring model: Management

- Nursing care appropriate
- Nursing care controversial
  (professional opinion varies regarding appropriate clinical management)
- Nursing care inappropriate
- Reviewer uncertain

Role of peer review in patient safety

Root-cause analysis vs. peer review

- Asking the system questions
- Reducing human error through system improvements
- Communicating lessons learned

Questions & Answers

Finally, provide plenty of opportunity for the audience to ask questions. Peer review is a complicated process for those unfamiliar with it, so remind the audience that no question is a stupid question.

Committee Members' Education

You can adapt the same PowerPoint to be used during training of the people who will sit on the peer review committee. When training committee members, it is helpful to include both a formal PowerPoint presentation at the beginning to help them begin the process and then follow up with ongoing education and working groups within the committee.

When conducting education of committee members, discuss issues of confidentiality, impartiality, and bias. A joint training session is a good idea to review the policy and expectations for the peer review process.

It is also imperative to discuss scoring. At the beginning, one of the biggest challenges that may be encountered by the committee is the actual scoring of cases. Committee members initially may approach scoring in different ways due to inexperience with the process. You may find that some committee members are much tougher than others. But it is important that all committee members reach consensus on scoring, and one way to achieve this is to conduct initial scoring of cases as a group so that the group learns to score the same way. It is crucial to ensure that scoring deviation does not occur between committee members.

For the first several meetings, committee members should all review the cases and score them together. The discussion that will ensue will educate the members regarding what cases are not appropriate for nursing peer review (e.g., cases that involve personality issues, such as a nurse shouting at a patient) and those cases that need to be referred for review by the medical staff.

Chapter 7

STEP 4

Implement the Nursing Peer Review Process

Learning objectives After reading this chapter, the participant will be able to:

- List the different components of the case review form
- Identify the essential step needed to achieve a standardized approach to scoring a case review form

Now that the formal policy, charter, process, and members of the committee have been established, you are probably wondering how to bring the program to fruition and start monitoring nursing performance on a continual basis.

Once the structure and processes have been established and everyone on the committee is trained and ready to begin, the first step is to determine if there is a case to review or to identify cases. In fact, some organizations may have a backlog of cases waiting for review and thus will have several cases to choose from. Using the list of predetermined review indicators identified by the organization can assist in choosing cases to forward through the case review process. For example, the organization may decide initially to keep it simple using data that are already collected and nurse specific. The following are some examples of indicators:

- Prevention of pressure ulcers
- Reduction of medication errors, which can be more specific, such as "omissions" or 5 medication rights
- Prevention of falls

- Completeness of documentation may include:
  - Nursing assessment within 24 hours
  - Medication reconciliation
  - Patient education at discharge
- Quality or patient safety concerns, such as adverse outcomes
- Policy compliance
- Patient satisfaction

Pick a Start Date to Implement the Program

While choosing a starting date may seem inconsequential, we highly recommended that you pick a specific date to begin the formal process of nursing peer review. Determining and communicating that specific date provides every nurse on staff with the same opportunity to start with a blank slate—from that day on, nurses know that everyone is held to the same standard.

If you have backlog of cases waiting for review, consider whether these cases are best for peer review or whether they should be dealt with in another manner. It may be best that some of these old cases proceed through the new format, based on their severity, but bear in mind that it can be difficult to go back in time and rehash old issues and concerns. Nurses may be resentful if past cases are dredged up, and this may harm the credibility of the process.

The start date should be established only after general nursing staff education is completed. The process will backfire if it is begun before nurses understand what to expect.

GO TO › Refer back to Chapter 6 for a step-by-step run through staff education

Conducting Chart Review

Practice makes perfect. This is as true with performing chart review as with anything else. In addition, peer review committee members have very different personalities and learning styles, so they may, at first, have different approaches to scoring a case. This is why it is helpful to score the first case—or few cases—together.

Achieving cohesiveness

Before the first meeting, all committee members should score the same case so that it may then be discussed during the first meeting. During the committee meeting, members can discuss any differences they had in the scoring process and come to an understanding on the best way to score cases.

Learning the process together and discussing issues as they come up will help the committee achieve cohesiveness and similarity in scoring and eliminate bias. Members on the committee will have the clinical knowledge to successfully perform a chart review, but they will need to practice using the new case scoring form to become comfortable and to ensure that all members of the committee approach the scoring in the same way.

Some organizations choose to create a fictional case for the first agenda meeting. This allows everyone to practice and discuss a case in complete freedom. However, the problem with dummy cases is that there is no medical record and no additional sources to back up the information and provide more detail. It is often easier to take a real case, score it beforehand, and then discuss during the meeting how everyone scored it. The first case will generate numerous questions; having additional information available can help resolve them.

Scoring the First Case

The nursing peer review case rating form is included in its entirety as Figure 7.1, but the form can be overwhelming when viewed as a whole, so we have broken it down into its composite sections so the different stages can be discussed. The rest of the chapter will discuss how to fill out the form.

FIGURE 7.1 | **Nursing peer review case rating form**

MR # __________ D/C date __________ Referral date ___________ Nurse Name/# _____________

Referral source: Check the corresponding box

❑ Screen ❑ Risk ❑ HIM ❑ Nursing ❑ Pharmacy ❑ Pt. Relations ❑ Med Staff ❑ Other _____

Review criteria/Referral issue: ____

Quality screener/Date: _______________ **Date submitted for nurse review:** _______________

Case summary: ____

____

____

____

____

Key issues for nurse reviewer: ____

____

____

____

To be completed by nurse reviewer

Nurse reviewer:____________________________________ Review date: _______________

Outcome: Check one		
	1	No adverse outcome
	2	Minor adverse outcome (complete recovery expected)
	3	Major adverse outcome (complete recovery **NOT** expected)
	4	Catastrophic adverse outcome (e.g., death)

Effect on patient care: Check one		
	1	Care not affected
	2	Increased monitoring/ observation (e.g., vital sign checks)
	3	Additional treatment/ intervention (e.g., IV fluids)
	4	Life sustaining treatment/ intervention (e.g., CPR)

FIGURE 7.1 **Nursing peer review case rating form (cont'd.)**

Overall nursing care: Check one		
	1	Appropriate
	2	Controversial
	3	Inappropriate
	0	Reviewer uncertain, needs committee discussion

Issue identification: Check all that apply		
	A	No issues with nursing care
Nursing care issues		
	B	Critical thinking
	C	Assessment
	D	Technique/skills
	E	Knowledge
	F	Communication
	G	Planning
	H	Follow-up/follow-through
	I	Policy compliance
	J	Supervision (nursing student)
	O	Other:

Note:
If overall care = 1, **then** issue must = (A);
If overall care = 2, 3, or 0,
then issue must = (B) through (O)

If overall nursing care rated 2, 3, or 0, give a **brief description** of the basis for reviewer findings or concerns:

____

____

____

____

____

If overall nursing care rated 2, 3, or 0, **what questions** are to be addressed by the nurse or the council?

____

____

____

____

____

FIGURE 7.1 **Nursing peer review case rating form (cont'd.)**

Nursing documentation: Check all that apply		
	1	No issue with nursing documentation
	2	Documentation does not substantiate clinical course and treatment
	3	Documentation not timely to communicate with other caregivers
	4	Documentation unreadable
	9	Other:

Documentation issue description: ____________________

____

Exemplary nominations: ❑ Nursing care ❑ Nursing documentation

Brief description: ____________________

Nonnursing care issues: ❑ Potential system or process issue ❑ Potential physican care issue

Issue description: ____________________

____

Committee review

Is nurse response needed? ❑ Yes ❑ No

Nurse response: ❑ Discussion with chair ❑ Letter ❑ Committee appearance

Committee final scoring:

Outcome: ____ Documentation: ____ Problem identification: ____ Overall nursing care: ____

Committee action: Check one		**Date completed**
	No action warranted	
	Nurse self-acknowledged action plan sufficient	
	Educational letter to nurse sufficient	
	Dept. manager discussion of informal improvement plan with nurse	
	Dept. manager develops formal improvement plan with monitoring	
	Refer to nursing leadership for formal corrective action	

FIGURE 7.1 **Nursing peer review case rating form (cont'd.)**

❑ System problem identified—forward to QCC

Date sent ______ Date response ______

Describe system issue ____

❑ Nursing standards issue—forward to nursing leadership

Date sent ______ Date response ______

Describe nursing concern ____

❑ Potential physician issue—forward to medical staff

Date sent __________

____

Nursing Peer Review Chair

Initial quality analyst screening

Figure 7.2 is the top section of the scoring form. This part of the form is filled out by the initial case quality analyst/screener prior to sending to a nurse reviewer on the committee.

FIGURE 7.2 **Case rating form—initial screening section**

MR # __________ D/C date ___________ Referral date ___________ Nurse Name/# ____________

Referral source: Check the corresponding box

❑ Screen ❑ Risk ❑ HIM ❑ Nursing ❑ Pharmacy ❑ Pt. Relations ❑ Med Staff ❑ Other _____

Review criteria/Referral issue: ____

Quality screener/Date: ____________________ **Date submitted for nurse review:** ____________

Case summary: ____

____

____

____

____

Key issues for nurse reviewer: ____

____

____

____

The quality analyst fills in the following parts of the top section of the scoring tool:

MR#: The patient's medical record number.

> **NOTE ›** For the purpose of confidentiality, the patient name is not included on the form.

D/C date: The date of patient's discharge from the hospital.

> **NOTE ›** There are instances that may occur when the patient is still in house and the case needs to be reviewed.

Referral date: The date that the case was referred for peer review and to be screened by the quality analyst/screener.

Nurse #: The primary nurse involved in the case (this can be tracked by name or by nurse ID number).

> **NOTE ›** In some instances, there may be more than one nurse involved in the case; create a separate review form and have a different nurse reviewer complete the case review.

Referral source: Where the referral came from.

Review criteria/referral issue: Peer review criteria established based on the referral issue (e.g., unanticipated death, medication administration error).

Quality analyst/screener, date: Person who performs initial screen of case and date the screen was completed.

Date submitted for nurse review: Date that quality screener submits case to the nurse reviewer on the committee.

Case summary: The quality screener writes a summary of the case as it pertains to the review criteria and that explains the referral issue—the summary should be brief for the nurse reviewer, not an exhaustive description of the case.

Key issues for nurse reviewer: This is an opportunity for the quality analyst/screener to highlight any other information that the nurse reviewer should focus on while reviewing the case.

Nurse reviewer

Once the top portion is filled out by the quality analyst/screener, the entire form and the case are submitted to a nurse reviewer on the committee. The nurse reviewer's responsibility is to review the case and make recommendations, and the nurse reviewer uses the next section of the case rating form, shown in Figure 7.3.

FIGURE 7.3 | **Case rating form—nurse reviewer section**

To be completed by nurse reviewer

Nurse reviewer:______________________________ Review date: ______________

Outcome: Check one		
	1	No adverse outcome
	2	Minor adverse outcome (complete recovery expected)
	3	Major adverse outcome (complete recovery **NOT** expected)
	4	Catastrophic adverse outcome (e.g., death)

Effect on patient care: Check one		
	1	Care not affected
	2	Increased monitoring/ observation (e.g., vital sign checks)
	3	Additional treatment/ intervention (e.g., IV fluids)
	4	Life sustaining treatment/ intervention (e.g., CPR)

Overall nursing care: Check one		
	1	Appropriate
	2	Controversial
	3	Inappropriate
	0	Reviewer uncertain, needs committee discussion

Issue identification: Check all that apply		
	A	No issues with nursing care
Nursing care issues		
	B	Critical thinking
	C	Assessment
	D	Technique/skills
	E	Knowledge
	F	Communication
	G	Planning
	H	Follow-up/follow-through
	I	Policy compliance
	J	Supervision (nursing student)
	O	Other:

Note:

If overall care = 1, **then** issue must = (A)

If overall care = 2, 3, or 0, **then** issue must = (B) through (O)

If overall nursing care rated 2, 3, or 0, give a **brief description** of the basis for reviewer findings or concerns:

____

____

____

FIGURE 7.3 **Case rating form—nurse reviewer section**

If overall nursing care rated 2, 3, or 0, **what questions** are to be addressed by the nurse or the council?

____

____

____

Nursing documentation: Check all that apply		
	1	No issue with nursing documentation
	2	Documentation does not substantiate clinical course and treatment
	3	Documentation not timely to communicate with other caregivers
	4	Documentation unreadable
	9	Other:

Documentation issue description: ____________________________

____

Exemplary nominations: ❑ Nursing care ❑ Nursing documentation

Brief description: ____________________________

Nonnursing care issues: ❑ Potential system or process issue ❑ Potential nursing care issue

Issue description: ____________________________

____

The nurse reviewer fills in the following areas:

Nurse reviewer: Name of the committee member who is to review the case.

Review date: Date that the nurse from the committee reviews the case.

Outcome: This box includes four descriptions based on the patient's outcome from which the nurse reviewer can report the patient's condition by checking one section from the following:

- No adverse outcome
- Minor adverse outcome
- Major adverse outcome
- Catastrophic adverse outcome (e.g., death)

Only one selection is needed in this category. Organizations should determine what constitutes minor, major, and catastrophic adverse outcomes as they create the structure and develop the committee. For example, minor adverse outcome is defined as complete recovery expected, major adverse outcome is when complete patient recover is not expected, and catastrophic adverse outcome results in patient death.

Effect on patient care: This box includes the effect that the nurse's care had on the patient's case or outcome. Only one of the following options should be selected:

- Care not affected
- Increased monitoring/observation
- Additional treatment/intervention
- Life-sustaining treatment/intervention

Issue identification: This box is where the nurse reports the issues that he or she identifies based on the nurse's care to the patient. This is an area where the reviewer can choose more than one issue. For example, the nurse reviewer may find that the nurse involved in a case had an assessment issue because the patient's blood pressure was dropping postprocedure and the nurse did not follow policy compliance by taking vital signs every 15 minutes postprocedure. Therefore, the reviewer would check both boxes, because both apply. Another example may be that a nurse did not call a physician regarding a critical lab value, which is once again a policy compliance issue and therefore also includes communication and follow-through issues. Categories of issues that may be identified by the nurse reviewer include:

- No issue with nursing care
- Critical thinking
- Assessment
- Technique/skill
- Knowledge
- Communication
- Planning
- Follow-up or follow-through
- Policy compliance
- Supervision (nursing student)
- Other

Overall nursing care: This box refers to the final determination of the case and the care rendered by the nurse involved. Reviewers must check one of the following options:

- Appropriate
- Controversial
- Inappropriate
- Reviewer uncertain, needs committee discussion

NOTE › If the issue selected in the issue identification box is "no issue," then the overall nursing care must be "care appropriate." Again, organizations must determine their own standards for what constitutes appropriate care. The nursing administration at the hospital is responsible for setting the appropriate nursing standards with guidance from state and federal rules and regulations.

Nursing documentation: This box is an area to identify any issues in the quality of the documentation. Reviewers are asked to check all applicable options for this section, including:

- No issue with nursing documentation
- Documentation does not substantiate clinical course and treatment
- Documentation not timely to communicate with other caregivers
- Documentation unreadable
- Other

NOTE › You may find cases that proceed through peer review that result in "care appropriate" determination but that issues with documentation were identified. This is a prime example of issues that organizations should be following and can track and trend data to identify whether individual nurses have documentation problems or concerns that should be monitored or dealt with proactively.

Exemplary nominations: The peer review process also encourages committees to recognize nurses for exemplary care or documentation. You will find that staff nurses at your organization will have a perception that peer review cases only ever identify poor care issues, but if nurses start receiving letters recognizing excellent care or documentation, then the image of the committee improves.

If in the course of a review the nurse reviewer or committee identifies exemplary issues, then these should be marked. A letter is sent to the nurse involved outlining the excellence in care or documentation.

GO TO › A sample letter documenting excellence is included as Figure 7.7 later in this chapter.

Nonnursing care issues: In the course of a review, the peer review committee may identify non-nursing issues that should be forwarded to the appropriate committee. For example, if a physician or system issue is identified, a letter should be sent from the nursing peer review committee to the physician peer review committee or to another appropriate entity. The nursing committee can ask for feedback and follow up on the issue so that it can "close the loop" on the case. Care should be taken, however, to make sure the nursing peer review committee does not waste time discussing physician care issues; circumstances out of the committee's scope should be immediately passed on to the appropriate place.

If a nonnursing care issue has been identified, the form should be completed by the nurse reviewer and scored in the overall nursing care section as "1: care appropriate." At this point, the case is then considered closed, and a letter is sent to the nurse involved in the case.

GO TO › You will find a template non-nursing issue letter in Figure 7.6.

The nurse is informed that a "care appropriate" determination has been made but not if a physician issue or any other issue has been identified. That is dealt with anonymously by the peer review committee.

When the nurse reviewers scores cases as "2: care controversial," "3: care inappropriate," or "0: reviewer uncertain," then the case will need committee discussion and should be placed on the next meeting agenda for discussion by the committee as a group.

The nurse reviewer may be assigned randomly or the nurse with the most appropriate clinical experience, such as a pediatric certified nurse reviewing a case involving a pediatric patient, may be chosen.

Drafting the First Agenda

The very first committee meeting may focus solely on committee members becoming acquainted, but for the first meeting involving case discussion, it is important to set an agenda so that the meeting will be structured and committee discussion can stay on track. Agendas should be created every time the committee meets.

The agenda should be presented in the same template for each committee meeting even if some sections don't have any items for discussion. Agendas should be retained by the quality analyst in a committee binder or as determined by the committee.

Figure 7.4 is a sample agenda that provides structure to the committee meeting and keeps the committee members focused on the committee goals.

FIGURE 7.4 **Nursing peer review sample agenda**

Agenda

Date: ______________________________

1. Call to order
2. Approval of minutes
3. Communications from other committees
   - Follow-up
   - New communications
4. Case reviews
   a) Rule indicators
      - Nursing or organizational policy

   b) Review indicators
      - Summary report of "care appropriate" cases
      - New case reviews requiring committee discussion
      - Follow-up on previous cases
      - Exemplary nominations

   c) Rate indicators
      - Nursing staff and department indicator trends requiring discussion
      - Nursing-specific rate indicator issues requiring discussion
5. Adjournment

Holding the First Meeting

At the committee meeting, the nurse reviewer who examined the case will discuss it in detail with the committee members and will share his or her issues and thoughts. Then the entire committee will engage in an open discussion about the case.

Committee meetings should be led by a chair appointed to keep the discussion on track and the meetings moving along as necessary.

NOTE › the committee chair does not normally complete case reviews on an ongoing basis due to oversight of committee responsibilities. It is best to schedule the meetings for no more than 90 minutes in length. Agenda items that are not covered can be tabled for the next committee meeting.

The final section of the case rating form, shown in Figure 7.5, is filled out by the quality analyst after the committee has discussed the case, as it includes the committee decision.

The following areas are to be populated, and the definitions are included below:

Is nurse response needed? Yes/No: If the committee agrees that the overall care rating is a "2" or "3," then a response from the nurse involved is warranted to explain the specific issues regarding the case.

Nurse response: The nurse involved in the case can respond to the committee either through discussion with the chair, by letter, or in person before the committee. If the committee determines that it would like the response in a letter format, the details of the case are outlined and the key questions that need to be answered are also included. Once a letter or response has been given to the committee by the nurse involved, the final scoring is then completed.

GO TO › A sample issue inquiry letter is included as shown in Figure 7.8.

Committee final scoring: This area captures the final scoring determination from the review portion of the form.

FIGURE 7.5 **Case rating form—committee review section**

Committee review

Is nurse response needed? ❑ Yes ❑ No

Nurse response: ❑ Discussion with chair ❑ Letter ❑ Committee appearance

Committee final scoring:

Outcome: ____ Documentation: ____ Problem identification: ____ Overall nursing care: ____

	Committee action: Check one	**Date completed**
	No action warranted	
	Nurse self-acknowledged action plan sufficient	
	Educational letter to nurse sufficient	
	Dept. manager discussion of informal improvement plan with nurse	
	Dept. manager develops formal improvement plan with monitoring	
	Refer to nursing leadership for formal corrective action	

❑ System problem identified—forward to QCC

Date sent __________ Date response __________

Describe system issue ______________________________

❑ Nursing standards issue—forward to nursing leadership

Date sent __________ Date response __________

Describe nursing concern ______________________________

❑ Potential physician issue—forward to medical staff Date sent __________

____

Nursing Peer Review Chair

Committee action: This box captures the final committee action for the case. Options are:

- No action warranted
- Nurse self-acknowledged action plan sufficient
- Educational letter to nurse sufficient
- Department manager discussion of informal improvement plan with nurse
- Department manager develops formal improvement plan with monitoring
- Refer to nursing leadership for formal corrective action

System problem identified: If a system problem is identified during the course of the review, then this area can be used to track where the problem was forwarded, the date it was forwarded, and when the committee received a response.

Nursing standard issue: If a nursing standard issue was identified during the course of the review, this area is used to track where the problem was forwarded, the date it was forwarded, and when the committee received a response back.

Potential physician issue: If a physician issue was identified during the course of the review, this area can be used to track where the problem was forwarded, the date it was forwarded, and when the committee received a response.

Discussing the case

As the committee discusses the case, members may decide immediately that the care provided was appropriate and issue a letter to the nurse involved informing him or her of the outcome.

Another option is that the committee may need more information before it can make a determination. Committees have the option of seeking advice from other people or experts—for example, they may ask a respiratory therapist to come before the committee and discuss usual standards of care in a given situation or discuss a lab value—so that they can better understand whether care in the real case deviated from usual practices.

If outside advisors are brought before the committee or their advice is solicited, no details about the case being discussed should be disclosed. It is imperative that the confidentiality of the peer review process always be maintained.

The committee may want to solicit further information from the nurse involved in the case, which can be done through letter, discussion with the chair or nurse reviewer, or in person before the committee. Each of these methods has advantages and disadvantages, such as the following:

1. **Requesting by letter.** The least intimidating option for the nurse being reviewed is to respond via letter. This means the committee must draft a letter asking specific questions and provide the nurse enough time to respond.
2. **Requesting a personal appearance before the committee.** Appearing before the committee can be an extremely stressful experience for the nurse involved as well as uncomfortable for committee members, who may be reluctant to ask all the questions they need answered.
3. **Requesting a one-on-one discussion.** A less intimidating option is for the chair to have a one-on-one discussion with the nurse, but that can also present problems. A one-on-one conversation makes the case a "he said, she said" issue and both parties may interpret the discussion differently. In addition, a conversation lacks documentation. If the one-on-one discussion is still the preferred method, you should have a third party in the room to act as a witness.

In fact, the preferred method is to send a letter, so that detailed questions may be noted and responded to with careful consideration.

Once the committee has completed its thorough discussion and is ready to make a decision, the easiest way to decide on a case is to take a vote. In rare occasions, there may be differences in the way committee members want to score a case, and committees should attempt to reach a consensus. It may be that they have not asked the right questions of the nurse involved, in which case follow-up questions may elicit answers. However, there may be times when the committee members cannot reach consensus, in which case it is helpful if the committee is composed of an uneven number of people. This way, the committee will never be split exactly in half on a decision.

The committee chair and the quality analyst are nonvoting members of the committee. If the committee ever reaches a point at which a decision cannot be made, the chair can break a tie in voting.

In the rare event that the committee is completely deadlocked on an issue and opinions are so divided that consensus cannot be reached, a last resort may be to seek external peer review—for example, from a sister hospital or a consultant. However, this is generally not recommended and should be considered only in the worst circumstances. Peer review should be an internal process, one that is conducted by the peers of the nurse being examined.

Final Determination

Once the committee has made a final determination, it may proceed in a number of ways. All involve documentation of the case and informing the nurse involved of what was concluded.

Care appropriate

Cases that are deemed "care appropriate" should still be reported back to the nurse, and the issue should be tracked.

A sample letter template is shown in Figure 7.6.

FIGURE 7.6 | **Letter: Care appropriate—no issue**

Dear Nurse ______________________,

The Nursing Peer Review Committee of the nursing staff reviewed the following case in which you were the nurse involved in the patient's care.

MR #: Discharge date:
Criteria for review:
Case summary:

The Committee concluded that there were no issues identified, either with nursing care or documentation, with regard to the care you provided to this patient. No follow-up activity is needed for this case.

This letter has been sent simply to inform you that your case was reviewed because the nursing staff wishes its members to be aware of all peer review activities involving their patients, regardless of the findings.

There is no need for you to respond. We thank you for the care that you provided to this patient.

Respectfully submitted,
Nursing Peer Review Committee

Exemplary care

Sending out letters praising and recognizing exemplary care or documentation is a rewarding part of the peer review committee and one that should be done whenever possible. Sending such letters helps improve the image of the committee, which, as we've discussed, many nurses believe exists solely for punitive reasons.

Recognizing when excellent care is performed will emphasize that the peer review committee is a positive committee. Peer review is not a "gotcha" process—it is about identifying exemplary care as much as it is about identifying and understanding care, documentation, or systems issues.

See Figure 7.7 for a sample exemplary plan letter you can adapt as needed.

FIGURE 7.7 **Letter: Care exemplary**

Dear Nurse ___________________________,

The Nursing Peer Review Committee of the nursing staff reviewed the following case in which you were the nurse involved in the patient's care.

MR #: Discharge date:
Criteria for review:
Case summary:

The Committee concluded that there were no issues identified, either with nursing care or documentation, with regard to the care you provided to this patient. No follow-up activity is needed for this case.

In the course of the review, the committee identified the following exemplary practice:

The Committee wishes to commend you for the care you provided for this patient.

This letter has been sent simply to inform you that your case was reviewed because the nursing staff wishes its members to be aware of all peer review activities involving their patients regardless of the findings. There is no need for you to respond. We thank you for the care that you provided to this patient.

Respectfully submitted,
Nursing Peer Review Committee

Further information

Letters sent to nurses to solicit further information and details about cases can be extremely useful in determining the correct outcome.

A sample issue inquiry letter is included as Figure 7.8.

FIGURE 7.8 **Letter: Issue inquiry**

Dear Nurse ______________________,

The Nursing Peer Review Committee of the nursing staff reviewed the following case in which you were the nurse involved in the patient's care.

MR #: Discharge date:
Criteria for review:
Case summary:

Based on the information available in the patient's medical record, the preliminary review of the case has raised the following questions:

We recognize the medical record often does not contain all the information needed to evaluate care in a complex case. Prior to the Committee making a determination on the case, we would like to have your input in writing to the above questions to more fully understand the care provided to this patient.

It is the policy of the nursing staff that this response is needed within 14 days of the receipt of this letter so the Committee can review cases in a timely fashion. If your response is not received in the appropriate time frame, unfortunately by policy, the committee will have to complete its evaluation without your valuable input.

If you have some mitigating circumstance that would preclude you from meeting this time frame, please contact your nursing supervisor immediately.

Respectfully submitted,
Nursing Peer Review Committee

Determination letter

Once the case has been finalized by the committee, a letter is sent to the nurse involved regarding the final determination of the case. This is also an opportunity for the committee to recommend whether a specific education/training session is needed for the involved nurse. A sample final determination letter is shown in Figure 7.9.

FIGURE 7.9 **Letter: Final determination**

Dear Nurse ______________________,

The Nursing Peer Review Committee of the nursing staff reviewed the following case in which you were the nurse involved in the patient's care.

MR #: Discharge date:
Criteria for review:
Case summary:

We thank you for your response to the Committee's questions regarding this case. However, based on the Committee's discussion, it concluded the following with regard to the care you provided to this patient:

Patient outcome:
Documentation:
Issues:
Overall physician care:

The basis for the Committee's conclusion was as follows:

In the spirit of nursing education and improvement, this letter has been sent to inform you of the Committee's conclusion. Based on the issues identified and your response, as a follow-up to this review, the Committee has recommended the following:

There is no need for you to respond to this letter. However, if you have any questions, please feel free to contact the Committee Chair.

Respectfully submitted,
Nursing Peer Review Committee

Peer review committees may be creative in their recommendations, such as recommending that the nurse attend a course on a particular issue. All the final determinations must be tracked and trended, which is discussed in Chapter 8, which explains how to use data from the peer review committee to monitor performance indicators.

Chapter 8

Track and Trend Your Data

PEER REVIEW AS A PERFORMANCE IMPROVEMENT TOOL

Learning objectives

After reading this chapter, the participant will be able to:

- Describe why it is important to track and trend data on a continual basis
- List the different types of indicators used to evaluate nursing performance

Peer review is about more than just case review—it is also about improving overall nurse performance. Peer review allows for the tracking and trending of data that has traditionally not been captured. Nursing has long captured clinical performance data by unit and specialty but traditionally not by individual nurse.

This chapter will demonstrate how to use peer review case outcomes, incidents of noncompliance, and rate-based data to track performance indicators. But first, we will discuss indicator types.

Measuring Performance and Understanding Indicator Types

Performance measures, also called indicators, do more than provide data; they indicate how something is actually performing. For example, the speedometer indicates how fast a car is going, and although a driver might have a general idea of speed from his or her own driving experience, using a speedometer is usually more objective. Similarly, nurses may have a good sense of another nurse's performance if they have worked with that nurse, but actually defining performance indicators provides a more objective way for nurses to evaluate each other.

There are two ways to classify performance indicators. The first is based on the classic Donabedian model of assessing quality of care, which is organized in terms of structure, process, and outcome. The second is based on three methods of analyzing performance: chart review, rule compliance, and rate-based outcomes data.

Donabedian Indicators

According to the classic Donabedian triangle (Donabedian 1996) (see Figure 8.1), you can assess the quality of nursing care by looking at information about structure, process, or outcome. The idea is that good structure increases the likelihood of good process and that good process increases the likelihood of good outcome. But knowing exactly what it is about structure, process, or outcome that is actually related to quality is no easy task, as we will discuss next.

FIGURE 8.1 | **Donabedian's quality triangle**

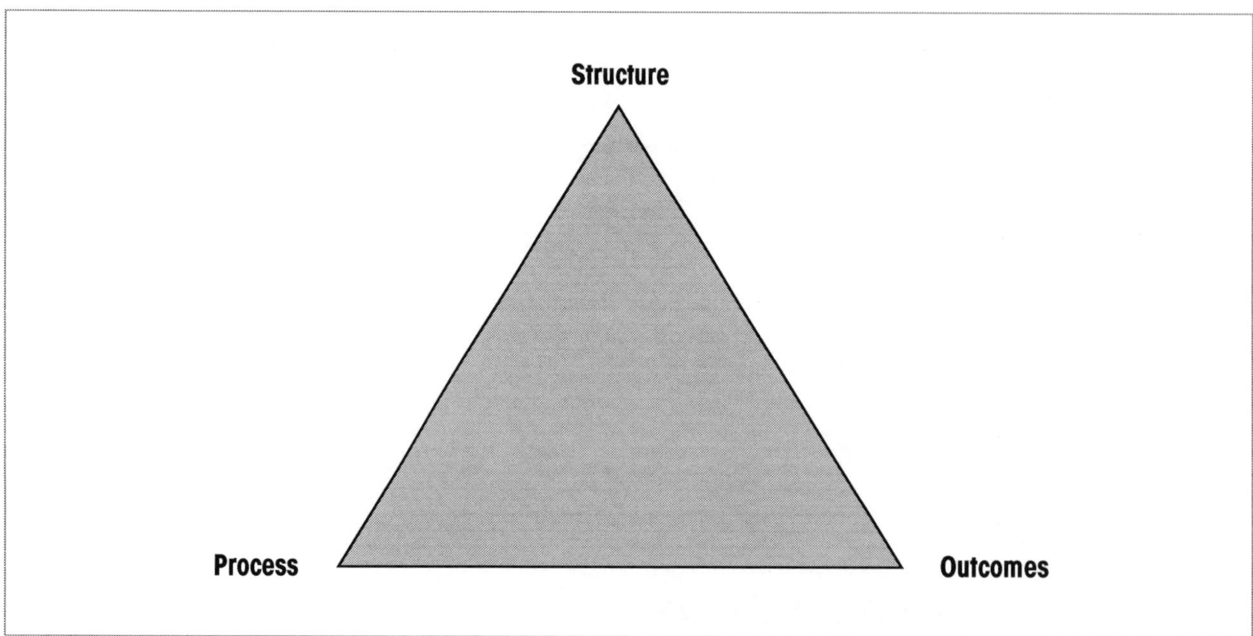

Structure indicators

Structure indicators examine the attributes of the setting in which care occurs. They include, for example, the qualifications of the care provider and the material resources available, such as facilities and equipment.

Consider the following question: Which hospital has the best chance of preserving an acute myocardial infarction (AMI) patient's myocardium: Hospital A, which offers only thrombolytic therapy, or Hospital B, which offers both thrombolytic therapy and interventional cardiac procedures? We can answer this question without even knowing how fast or how well the cardiac intervention could be performed. That's because we know that not all AMI patients qualify for thrombolytics and that studies have shown that interventions such as angioplasty and placing intraarterial stents will preserve myocardium. Thus, because Hospital B has a particular capability, or structure, an AMI patient treated there is more likely to have a better outcome.

Structure indicators are easy to obtain. However, when assessing the potential value of a structure indicator, you must determine whether it is, in fact, related to quality. We must not accept structural measures that are based on untested assumptions. For example, a common structural measure is nursing certification, but "proof" of past clinical competency does not measure how a nurse practices today. Although there now appears to be evidence of a general relationship between nursing certification and the quality of nursing care, the widespread use of this structure indicator began well before those data were available.

Many such regulatory structure indicators of quality, often called standards, lack true correlation with quality, especially those developed by field consensus rather than by prospective studies. Still, until those data are available, those obliged to measure quality have to rely, at least in part, on structure indicators.

Process indicators

Process refers to how nurses deliver care. For example, a good process indicator for an intensive care unit (ICU) available at Hospital B would be the time it takes to respond to ICU critical alarms. Why? Because clinical studies show that the faster the response is, the better the quality of care as defined by ICU standards. And although performing a process well does not guarantee good quality, it is more closely associated with quality than is simply meeting a structure indicator.

But why measure process and not just measure the outcomes? One reason is that measuring a process is often easier because it occurs in the present and at the hospital. An outcome, on the other hand, may occur at some distant time or place. For example, because of short hospital stays, inpatient surgical wound infections often are not detected until after patients are discharged. However, studies show that timely preoperative prophylactic antibiotics reduce infection, so measuring the performance of the process of giving timely prophylactic antibiotics gives a good indication of the likelihood of fewer infections.

Unfortunately, as with structure indicators, it is easy to measure all kinds of processes, and hospitals sometimes do so just to show they have data on quality. But there should be reasonable evidence of a process outcome relationship before measuring a process—simply assuming the connection is not enough.

> **NOTE ›** Good process indicators measure processes that link to the desired outcome.

Outcome indicators

Outcome refers to what actually happens to the patient. Outcome indicators ask, "Did we really improve health? Did we heal? Did we avoid harm?"

Also note that although outcome indicators often are discussed in terms of clinical outcomes, it is important to consider resource outcome indicators, such as length of stay. Outcome indicators, however, can be difficult to measure, so it is important to focus on the right ones. Many outcome indicators today are being defined by medical specialties, payers, regulators, the government, and consumers, but remember that the reason behind giving nurses outcome data is so that they can use it to improve their performance.

The way to improve performance (i.e., the outcome) is to improve the process that produced the outcome. Therefore, although outcome indicators are the end goal, they must be reasonably linked to processes that can actually be improved.

Selecting process and outcome indicators

The best rule to apply when selecting outcome or process measures is to be sure that the process is linked to a known outcome that you want to improve and that the outcome is linked to a known process. That way, the nurses know what to improve. Sometimes you may wish to measure both process and outcome on the same performance area, because even though it may be easy to measure the outcome, intervention might occur earlier if you also measure the process.

Identifying Nursing Indicators

The main focus of this book is the peer review process and how to examine individual incidents, but organizations would be missing half of the value of peer review if they do not use the information generated to monitor nursing performance. This allows organizations to track data back to individual nurses and identify trends or patterns over time, allowing for intervention and correction. It serves as a mechanism to identify educational needs of the nurses as well.

The peer review process creates an opportunity to select, classify, and then monitor individual nursing performance over time. The way this is done is by selecting performance-based indicators, classifying the indicator type, and then managing nurse performance when an outlier has been reached.

But first, indicators have to be established. Selecting indicators based on nursing performance can be done by considering two key issues:

1. Consider what types of indicator data may be required either by federal, state-based, or accreditation entities. These are the easiest to select because they are a required indicator and you may already be collecting data sets.
2. Identify what types of data can be collected on an individual nurse basis (i.e., some data sets may be nurse relevant but you are not able to tag it to an individual because care is given by many nurses who may have contributed to the event).

Organizations will often find that data are being captured in areas around the organization on an aggregate basis, either by unit or specialty. But the questions to ask are "Is it possible to capture data on an individual basis?" and "How difficult is it to get to those data?"

This is the perfect time to create a list of all the indicator data sets currently being collected within the organization for nursing performance, such as medication errors, pressure ulcers, etc. The list of indicators used to monitor nursing performance should be categorized into columns with the following headings:

- Indicator name
- Indicator group (the nursing service for which the indicator is relevant)
- Indicator type (activity, review, rate, and rule)
- Nurse relevant/nurse specific
- Acceptable target
- Excellence target
- Data source

Once the indicator list has been generated, you can classify each indicator into four main types: activity, review, rule, and rates.

1. Activity indicators

Activity indicators are data sets that reflect a number or volume. For example, this may include number of patient encounters or number of medications administered by a nurse. This type of data can also be used as the denominator in rate-based indicators. The collection of activity data for this specific type of indicators can be abstracted from an existing system that is currently used in the facility or manually collected.

2. Review indicators

This type of indicator identifies a significant event that would ordinarily require analysis by nurse peers to determine cause, effect, and severity. Examples include all the screening criteria for peer review.

Examples of review indicators are shown in Figure 8.2.

FIGURE 8.2 | **Examples of review indicators**

Indicator group	Indicator	Indicator type	Nurse relevant	Nurse specific	Excellence target	Acceptable target	Data source
All nursing	Unanticipated death	Review	Yes	Yes	N/A	N/A	Referral and/or general screen
All nursing	Medication administration error	Review	Yes	Yes	N/A	N/A	Referral and/or pharmacy log
All nursing	Patient seen/not documented on a timely basis	Review	Yes	Yes	N/A	N/A	Referral

There are no target values for review-based indicators. Only the final determination outcomes of peer review cases are used to determine whether an individual has reached an outlier.

Measurement of review indicators

Outlined in the peer review policy are the thresholds for the peer review process specific to case review. These thresholds (i.e., benchmarks) will determine when a specific nurse has reached the outlined number of cases that then trigger an improvement plan.

GO TO › Refer to Chapter 5, Figure 5.1 for a copy of the peer review policy.

Therefore, suitable nurse indicators in regard to the peer review process could be the number of cases deemed controversial and number of cases deemed inappropriate. These two indicators are technically classified as "rule" indicators, but they are the aggregates of the peer review case outcomes.

The committee should determine thresholds for nurses concerning how many incidents are dealt with by the peer review committee in a given year. The threshold may be zero incidents in a year, which would receive an "excellent" rating. An "acceptable" threshold is two incidents in a year. Thus, anything more than that is considered and outlier and would trigger further examination. If a nurse were to have three cases in a one-year time frame, this would trigger a more focused review of the nurse's overall care.

3. Rule indicators

This type of indicator represents a general rule, standard, or generally recognized professional guideline or accepted practice of nursing where individual variation does not directly cause adverse patient outcomes. Ideally, there should always be compliance with "rules," but rare or isolated deviations from a rule usually represent only a minor problem.

If a rule event occurs, a "rule" letter is generated and sent to the nurse involved. A copy of the letter is maintained in a nurse file for such future reference as may be necessary. A target number of events should be set for each indicator based on the criticality of the rule to determine whether further follow-up is needed. If a pattern of rule events or a potentially serious isolated event is identified, it is reported to the nursing peer review committee as well as the appropriate department supervisor, who shall decide how to proceed.

Examples of rule indicators are shown in Figure 8.3.

FIGURE 8.3 | **Examples of rule indicators**

Indicator group	Indicator	Indicator type	Nurse relevant	Nurse specific	Excellence target	Acceptable target	Data source
All nursing	# of cases deemed "care inappropriate"	Rule	Yes	Yes	0/yr	2/yr	Manually collected
All nursing	Absence or presence of pain is not documented on all inpatients	Rule	Yes	Yes	0/yr	4/yr	Case Management
All nursing	Noncompliance with completion of standing orders	Rule	Yes	Yes	0/yr	3/yr	Case Management
All nursing	Validated incidents of nursing inappropriate behavior	Rule	Yes	Yes	0/yr	1/yr	Referral

Measurement of rule indicators

For rule indicators, targets are set based on the number of events or incidents of noncompliance to the specific rule. Rule indicator targets should be expressed in number of events over a given period of time. An example may be "less than four events every 12 months."

There are no external benchmarks for rule indicators, so the nursing staff and hospital should determine their own targets based on the performance levels for the specific rule that are acceptable to them, as well as to historical compliance levels. The more critical a rule is for compliance, the lower the target levels. For example, noncompliance with completion of standing orders should have a very small occurrence: zero per year would be deemed as excellent; two per year would be acceptable; greater than two per year would require intervention.

4. Rate indicators

This type of indicator identifies cases or events that are aggregated for statistical analysis prior to review by the appropriate committee or administrative function. This type of indicator may be expressed as a percentage, average, percentile rank, index, or ratio.

A target range should be established for each rate indicator, which may be based on best practice from benchmark data, statistical variation from the average, or internal targets.

Individual nurses should be provided with feedback on their rates on a regular and timely basis. If the rate for a particular nurse falls outside of the target range, the leadership of the appropriate nursing service would determine what, if any, action is warranted. Examples of rate indicators are shown in Figure 8.4.

FIGURE 8.4 **Examples of rate indicators**

Indicator group	Indicator	Indicator type	Nurse relevant	Nurse specific	Excellence target	Acceptable target	Data source
All nursing	% AMI patients receiving aspirin at arrival	Rate	Yes	Yes	95%	100%	Core measure vendor
All nursing	% compliance with nursing documentation	Rate	Yes	Yes	95%	100%	Manually collected
All nursing	Patient satisfaction with nursing care	Rate	Yes	Yes	90%	100%	Pt. satisfaction vendor

Measurement of rate indicators

Rate-based indicators measure the number of events that have occurred compared to the number of opportunities that the event could have occurred (i.e., numerator and denominator, respectively). Targets for rate indicators can be displayed as a percentage, average, index, ratio, etc. When you create rate-based indicators, make sure that the indicator description matches the data outcome.

For example, if percent of nursing compliance with documentation is 50 charts out of 120 medical records, then the percent of compliance is 42% (i.e., 50/120 = 0.41666 x 100 = 41.6%, rounded up to 42%).

Use external benchmarks (e.g., normative databases and literature) for targets whenever possible. In general, the distribution of the targets for rate indicators need not be symmetrical and can have a greater proportion of nurses in the "excellent" category than in the "needs follow-up" category.

Benchmarking and Using Performance-Based Data

Once data has been collected, tracked, and trended by individual nurses, there needs to be a way to use the data to monitor performance over time and to effect change. One of the most effective ways to monitor performance is by distributing data to the individual nurses on a regular basis. This can be done on a quarterly, biannual, or annual basis. This also allows nursing administration the ability to monitor performance over time.

If a nurse were to reach an outlier status for any indicator, then an improvement plan should be created to identify some key areas that may be the underlying or overlying factors. Key areas to consider when creating an improvement plan include:

1. Is the outlier status due to the acceptable and excellence target values being set too high or too low?
2. Is there something in regard to a standard protocol, procedure, or policy that may have affected how that nurse delivered care and thus created the outlier?
3. Does the nurse need additional mentoring based on the indicator and the outlier?

Improvement plans should be created by the nursing leadership team. For different types of indicators, the improvement plans may be different. For example:

1. Nurse Jones reaches an outlier for the rule indicator in regard to the peer review process: "number of cases deemed care inappropriate." The improvement plan may be that a focused 50 chart review is completed by a team of three or four nurses for a specific time frame. This focused review will look at all aspects of the nurse's care that was delivered.
2. Nurse Smith reaches an outlier for the rule indicator "absence or presence of pain is not documented on inpatients." The improvement plan may be to have a meeting with the nursing supervisor, the chair of the nursing peer review committee, and the nurse involved to discuss documentation requirements and provide additional education on the EMR if needed.

Reference

Donabedian, A. "Evaluating the quality of medical care." *Milbank Memorial Fund Quarterly* 44, no. 3 (Jul. 1996 Suppl.): 166–206.

Chapter 9

Using Data to Drive Improvement

CREATING A COMPREHENSIVE FEEDBACK REPORT

Learning objectives

After reading this chapter, the participant will be able to:

- Determine where indicator data are housed and how to extract it
- Identify different types of feedback reports
- Determine what the next steps are to improve performance when there are outliers based on data outcomes

Creating a nursing feedback report can be a challenge, but the advantages provided by performance analysis across the group far outweigh the effort you'll invest on the road to designing your report. Ultimately, the reports will be part of a system providing quantifiable data you can use to understand and address nursing performance throughout the team, unit, or even across the health system itself.

The process of collecting, analyzing, and disseminating the types of data discussed within this chapter differs from that followed by HR in evaluating for nursing privileges. The nursing peer review process requires a more defined and uniform use of measures (indicators) to assess nursing competency, above and beyond the hospital's formal HR process.

Before you begin the design of your comprehensive feedback report, however, you must seek out the answers to two deceptively simple-sounding questions. This chapter will guide you through the process of answering them as a way of establishing your report parameters.

Finding, Capturing, and Using Data

The answers to two simple questions will tell you how much and what type of effort will be involved in collecting data from existing sources, what kind of additional data you will need to collect, and how you will need to design the program to provide the most informative reporting format based on your chosen indicators.

1. **Where are the data?**

The first question is "Where do the data come from for each indicator?" Some data may be already gathered on an ongoing basis, by one or another group within the organization. Some may not.

2. **How will we manage and monitor nurse performance on an ongoing basis?**

Effective peer review is not only about measuring competency; it is also about managing and monitoring the data to improve patient care.

Availability of Indicator Data

Knowing what data sets are available can be a challenge; your first and arguably most important job is to identify the types of data sets that are already being captured in the hospital.

Most data are collected on a hospital, unit, or department level. A small amount of these data will be available at the nurse-specific level of granularity. Nurse-specific core measures are not often assigned to a nurse simply because the individuals charged with abstracting the data haven't been instructed to abstract the data sets with those identifiers. Additionally, more than one nurse takes care of a patient over a 24-hour period, making it difficult to assign a specific nurse when the event occurred. Often, the relevant measure is being collected for an aggregate data outcome or is being abstracted by a physician.

The key to determining whether nurse-specific data are available is to drill down into the details of how the data are being obtained. While the data sets may represent an aggregate for reporting purposes, deep within the data you may find the pot of gold—individual identifiers that you can use as you build your nursing peer review database.

Attribution of Data

One of the biggest concerns of collecting data on an individual nurse basis is verifying and maintaining the accuracy of *attribution*. It is critical that data sets are attributed to the correct nurse if they are to be used to improve individual nurse performance. Accurate attribution is paramount if you are to use data fairly in the peer review process.

Data collected on an individual basis typically uses a unique identifier. If any of the data systems in your organization use such a defined identifier for each nurse, your task of data collection will be somewhat easier. If not, you will have to collect the data manually to ensure that the data sets used in feedback reports are assigned to the right individual.

CAUTION › One of the biggest downfalls of displaying inaccurate data is that you risk losing the support of the entire nursing staff. The credibility of your peer review process will be in jeopardy.

Data Systems Inventory

Start by assessing your organization's ability to collect data. Using the defined list of nursing-specific indicators can guide you in the process of determining where data resides.

In most hospitals, the most centralized data source is the billing system. Unfortunately, patient care episodes are not billed by nursing, so other systems will need to be utilized to abstract nursing data. There are multiple data systems that are used throughout the organization in individual departments. Many hospitals have department/specialty databases that are not linked with the quality department and potentially could have nurse specific-data.

Working with the quality department to explore the many systems utilized in the hospital is very beneficial. The goal is to try to collect most data electronically; unfortunately, there will be a large number of data sets that are manually collected.

Feedback Report Formats

Once you have identified all your indicator data sources and systems, you are ready to create a comprehensive feedback report for each nurse on staff. As discussed in Chapter 2, we recommend using dimensions of performance to monitor nurse outcomes. Defining those dimensions of performance is also the first step in designing your feedback report.

Indicators and their descriptions are classified within a dimension of performance.

Dimensions of performance

1. Technical quality of care
2. Patient safety and rights
3. Quality of service

4. Resource utilization
5. Peer-to-coworker relationships
6. Contributions to hospital and community

Keep in mind that you do not need to use these specific dimensions of performance. If you currently have a framework for competency within the organization, by all means use it. Alternatively, the nursing staff as a whole may choose to create the framework or you may choose to use the existing peer review committee to establish the framework, dimensions, and format for your feedback reports.

Finding the Perfect Fit

You may find that in your organization the nursing performance data are not maintained in a database that produces easy-to-use reports. If you find yourself in this position, the hospital must decide to either design, purchase, or adapt an existing system to collect and produce reports with nurse-specific data. Even though accreditation and best practices would favor the use of a comprehensive feedback report, there is no rule to tell you that you must do so. In that sense, you have great flexibility in designing your report.

The design process must take into account how the reports will fit into the current nurse culture and help lead the existing culture toward better use of performance data. To accomplish this goal, the organization must assign the staff and resources to manage the database. Whether purchasing a system or building from scratch, the organization must:

1. **Select the database that best suits its purpose.** This may mean going through a request-for-proposals process to gather the pros and cons of the database.
2. **Select, implement, and continuously revise and update queries and reports.** This means pilot testing the report with a key group of nurses prior to rolling it out to the general nursing staff.

Feedback Report Formats

In designing the feedback report; the first step is to organize the indicators by the dimensions of performance. For nurses to understand which competency an indicator measures, it is important to organize the data by competency.

FIGURE 9.1 **Sample nurse feedback report**

Nurse Performance Feedback Report						
Nurse: Smith, Nancy	**Unit: Medicine**		**Time period: 2015 Qtr 1**			
Activity data						
Patient encounters						
# of committee meetings attended						
Performance data	**Indicator type**	**Numerator**	**Denominator**	**Excellence target**	**Acceptable target**	**Final score**
Technical quality						
# of case reviews deemed "care inappropriate"	Rule	1		0/yr	2/yr	Yellow
# of case reviews deemed "care controversial" or "inappropriate"	Rule	0		0/yr	4/yr	Green
# of cases with documentation issues identified by peer review	Rule	6		0/yr	5/yr	Red
Absence or presence of pain is not documented on all inpatients	Rule	0		0/yr	4/yr	Green
% AMI patients receiving aspirin at arrival	Rate	10	10	100%	95%	Green
Service quality						
Noncompliance with completion of standing orders	Rule	2		0/yr	3/yr	Yellow
Patient safety						
% compliance with nursing documentation	Rate	10	10	100%	95%	Green
Patient satisfaction with nursing care	Rate	0	2	100%	90%	Red
Validated incidents of patient not seen and/or documented daily by nurse	Rule	0		0/yr	2/yr	Green
Illegible medication order	Rule	3		2/yr	6/yr	Yellow
Peer to coworker relationships						
Validated incidents of inappropriate nurse behavior	Rule	0		0/yr	2/yr	Green
Resource utilization						

FIGURE 9.2 | **Explanation of feedback report format**

Explanation of Feedback Report Format

The sample feedback report format in Figure 9.1 contains the elements described below. The data and targets are illustrative examples and are not based on actual data.

Activity data: The amount of work by indicator done by the nurse.

Performance data: Measures of nurse data either using outcome or process indicators. In this column, the indicators should be listed by nurse dimension (e.g., Technical Quality, Service Quality, etc.).

Indicator type: Rule or rate. Peer review case outcomes are displayed as an aggregate rule indicator.

Numerator: # of incidents or occurrences.

Denominator: Total volume used to calculate the outcome vs. the numerator.

Excellence target: The threshold or target that separates excellent performance from acceptable performance.

Acceptable target: The threshold that separates acceptable performance from performance requiring follow-up.

Final score: The color or symbol indicating the relationship of the nurses' data to the targets for that indicator.

Separate activity data from performance data

Nursing activity data should be separated from performance data so as not to give the allusion that the hospital is evaluating activity. *Activity data* describes how much work a nurse completes within a given period. *Performance data* indicates how well a nurse does in his or her work. Lumping these two types of data sets together is not very useful in monitoring nurse performance. Keep in mind that activity data are not held to a specific benchmark or target.

Incorporating indicators, targets, and outcomes

Below the activity data, the indicators, targets, and outcomes will be displayed in a simple yet comprehensive format, as shown in Figure 9.3. Vendors use multiple types of formats to display data outcomes. We recommend that you select the method that the hospitals already uses (color codes) or create a new methodology that seems most effective and understandable.

FIGURE 9.3 **Indicator/outcomes display**

Nurse Feedback Report

Nurse: Smith, Nancy RN **ID:** 116 **Category:** Active **Unit/Specialty:** Medicine

Activity

Time period	ID#	Indicator title	Volume
3 Mo End 2014 Qtr 1	1	# of patient encounters	23
3 Mo End 2014 Qtr 1	74	# of committee meetings attended	3

Technical quality

Time period	ID#	Indicator title	Indicator type	Numerator			Acceptable value	Excellence value	Score
3 Mo End 2014 Qtr 1	4	# of cases with documentation issues identified by peer review	Rule	0			5	0	Green
3 Mo End 2014 Qtr 1	5	# of cases deemed care controversial	Rule	2			2	0	Yellow
3 Mo End 2014 Qtr 1	6	# of cases deemed inappropriate	Rule	1			2	0	Yellow
3 Mo End 2014 Qtr 1	8	Absence or presence of pain is not documented on all inpatients	Rule	4			3	1	Red
3 Mo End 2014 Qtr 1	61	% AMI patients receiving aspirin at arrival	Rate	3	3	100.0%	80.0%	95.0%	Green

Service Quality

Time period	ID#	Indicator title	Indicator type	Numerator			Acceptable value	Excellence value	Score
3 Mo End 2014 Qtr 1	84	Noncompliance with completion of standing orders	Rule	0			2	0	Green

Peer Review: Confidential Information *Saturday, August 30, 2014*

Nurse Manager____________ Date ____________

FIGURE 9.3 **Indicator/outcomes display (cont'd.)**

Contribution to Hospital & Community

Patient Safety

Time period	ID#	Indicator title	Indicator type	Numerator			Acceptable value	Excellence value	Score
3 Mo End 2014 Qtr 1	17	Validated incidents of patient not seen and/or documented daily by nurse	Rule	3			3	0	Yellow
3 Mo End 2014 Qtr 1	18	# of illegible medication orders	Rule	1			4	1	Green
3 Mo End 2014 Qtr 1	31	% patient satisfaction with nursing care	Rate	0	2	0.0%	90.0%	100.0%	Red

Peer to Coworker Relationships

Time period	ID#	Indicator title	Indicator type	Numerator			Acceptable value	Excellence value	Score
3 Mo End 2014 Qtr 1	16	# of validated incidents of inappropriate nurse behavior	Rule	1			3	0	Yellow

Resource Utilization

Peer Review: Confidential Information

Nurse Manager__________ Date __________

Saturday, August 30, 2014

Preparing and distributing feedback reports

Once you've completed the format design for your nursing feedback report, you are ready to bring the report to life. However, don't circulate it prematurely.

Many times, organizations apply pressure to get a feedback report out quickly, before the results have been thoroughly tested. If you succumb to this pressure, you will pay for it in the long run, because mistakes are bound to come to the surface.

Keep in mind, though, that the first report that is distributed doesn't have to be perfect or include data on all the dimensions of performance. Use the crawl, walk, run approach to getting started and keeping the momentum moving forward.

NOTE › The bottom line: Verify that your report is sound and functional. Refinements can be made over time.

Pilot test your design

Designing a pilot test need not be a complicated endeavor. This test will provide valuable information to make final adjustments before sending the report out to the masses.

The goal of your pilot test is to ensure that what you have designed is bias-free and understood by all. The following are a few options for selecting a pilot test group:

1. A single or a few units or departments
2. Members of a current nursing staff committee
3. A sample of nurses from each major unit or specialty

Once you have determined how to pilot test the feedback tool, the next step is to bring the group together. Bringing the group together to provide feedback is helpful—it provides a means for evaluating whether the tool is comprehensive and understood by all.

After distributing the feedback tool to the group, the next step is to ask some focused questions.

Go through each part of the report and define the data captured and/or fields of information. As questions arise, record them so that you can address further enhancements before implementation. You may also want to create a glossary of terms to assist in the educational process when implementing the feedback tool.

Although you may be tempted to start with a single unit because you only expect to create one type of report, this approach will limit the feedback you receive and the ultimate distribution of the report across the entire nursing staff. Working with a sample of nurses from different units or specialties is often a more effective and efficient way to get a broad view of your pilot test.

Managing performance with outcomes

The feedback reports have been developed, the pilot test has been completed, and the reports have been rolled out to the general nursing staff. So what is the next step? Using the data outcomes to improve performance.

In Chapter 8, we discussed creating indicators and setting targets or benchmarks to calculate outcomes. Each indicator is given an excellence and acceptable target. This is the data outcome range in order to determine what next steps will be taken.

- If a data outcome is excellence, the outcome is green. No further action is needed on this indicator data set.
- If the outcome falls below excellence but above acceptable, the outcome is yellow. This outcome is still considered to be satisfactory.
- If the outcome is below acceptable, the outcome is red.

Outcomes are discussed with the peer review committee and then an action plan is created. The action plan could consist of a meeting with the nurse/unit manager, an intensive chart review to look for patterns in practice, or additional nursing education sessions. Action plans can be different for different types of indicators and outcomes. (For example, you wouldn't create the same action plan for "noncompliance with standing order sets" and "validated incidents of inappropriate behavior.")

As you might guess, some of the actions are focused on systems rather than the nurse. It might be that a policy was created a decade ago and seemed reasonable at the time, but as time and processes change, we need to modify to bring it back to the standard. Discussing any such potential changes with nursing leaders is critical to determine the best process for the organization based on culture.

CAUTION > It is more important to take each step and implement it slowly than to rush and meet barriers that will be difficult to overcome.

Now that the essential components have been discussed on building a peer review program, it is time to take this step-by-step process and determine how to implement within your organization. Every organization is different, and while some can move quickly, others may not. Creating a timeline is often helpful and will allow the organization to implement the process over time. This will take months, and it often takes up to one year to implement all components with existing resources. The time is now for the nursing profession to hold itself accountable for the quality of nursing care and to understand the impact of care on the patient outcome.

Chapter 10

External Factors

ANCC MAGNET RECOGNITION PROGRAM® AND NURSING UNIONS

Learning objectives

After reading this chapter, the participant will be able to:

- Explain how a professional peer review process supports the 14 Forces of Magnetism
- Identify five steps to building trust with healthcare bargaining units or unions when conducting case-based nursing peer review

Now that you have a good grasp of the case-based peer review process, it is important to think about the future of your organization and the future direction for acute care hospitals in general. Consider the following questions:

- What external factors will influence a decision to implement peer review?
- What will our future hold in healthcare?
- What external agencies will have more power to regulate healthcare?
- What is the right time to implement a peer review program?

To have a successful peer review program, you'll develop a work plan incorporating peer review to meet the goals of your organization. In doing so, you may have to consider serving the goals of external organizations.

Some considerations, such as becoming an ANCC Magnet Recognition Program® (MRP) hospital, are choices that we can voluntarily pursue in the current healthcare environment. Other considerations, such as having nursing unions, will be factors we have no choice but to consider when crafting our nursing peer review process.

This chapter discusses the importance of the MRP standards and how to comply with them. It also provides guidance for how to obtain buy-in in a unionized environment.

ANCC Magnet Recognition Program®

Peer review and nursing excellence

As a process devoted to improving nurse performance and encouraging nurses to be accountable for their practice, peer review is a natural fit for many organizations pursuing MRP designation, which recognizes facilities that have achieved a high standard of nursing excellence.

Origins of the ANCC Magnet Recognition Program®

Research was conducted in the early 1980s to identify what hospital characteristics were associated with improved patient outcomes and higher quality. Hallmark studies by Margaret L. McClure, Marlene Kramer, Claudia Schmalenberg, and Linda Aiken found common characteristics among many high-performing nursing departments. Hospitals with the ability to attract and retain nurses, in a context of a professional environment, were called "magnet" hospitals because nurses were attracted to them and stayed with them.

The ANCC created a formal program to recognize hospitals as centers of nursing excellence and designated its first MRP organization in 1994. Since then, more than 400 hospitals have been designated as MRP facilities.

Integral components for an MRP environment are nursing leadership, professional models, and organizational structures that support and encourage autonomy, nursing excellence, and a strong sense of nursing identity and professionalism. Many designated hospitals find that over time the structures become almost invisible as the designation environment becomes a way of life rather than a goal.

MRP-designated facilities are those that disseminate, engage, and sustain all the 14 Forces of Magnetism and create an environment of quality outcomes for both patients and professional nurses.

Forces of Magnetism relating to peer review

Implementing peer review will provide compliance for the following three Forces of Magnetism: Force 4, Force 6, and Force 9. Working within the ANCC structure adds value to your program and certainly provides a model that drives excellence in nursing.

Force of Magnetism 4: Personnel Policies and Programs and Force of Magnetism 9: Autonomy both define areas that are applicable for the peer review process.

Force of Magnetism 4 refers to "formal, informal, regular and ongoing performance appraisal processes [which include] peer review" (ANCC, 2014), and Force 9 includes a description of "how the peer review process is used for professional growth for nurses at all levels in the organization" (ANCC, 2014).

Force of Magnetism 6: Quality of Care can also be readily applied to peer review for ensuring the "quality infrastructure . . . and the involvement of nurses from various settings and at all levels of the organization in establishing, monitoring, and evaluating practice standards."

Whether your hospital is thinking about this journey or not, applying the peer review principles will positively impact the patient safety culture in the hospital. You do not need to pursue MRP designation today, but it is something you may consider for the future.

Regardless, we recommend that you implement your peer review sooner rather than later.

Nursing Unionized Environments

Relationship

You may ask how it is possible to implement case-based peer review into a unionized environment. An obvious concern is that the union will see peer review as a punitive process designed to provide a means to terminate a nurse for poor performance.

The fact is that peer review provides information to nurses so that they can adjust their performance toward best practice, ultimately having a positive impact on patient care.

Different hospitals have different relationships with unions. In some cases, the relationship is solid, collegial in nature, and one of trust, which means that implementing peer review will not be difficult. On the other end of the spectrum, relationships that lack trust, are always in arbitration, and exist in a state of conflict are less likely to support the idea of nursing peer review. So the question is: How do you overcome the barriers, achieve buy-in, and manage the process to a successful outcome?

Open and honest communication provides the most important foundation for building trust with nursing unions. The dialogue between the two parties must focus on the patient first. For example, you might ask: What is in the best interest of the patient? Building trust and a collegial relationship can be difficult, especially if there has been a disconnect (or worse, conflict) for many years. So tread lightly and evaluate the relationship before implementing peer review.

> **CAUTION >** Timing is everything. It is far better to start with building the relationship as a first step in implementing peer review than to create your structure and meet resistance.

The approach to buy-in

The first step is to sit with the chief nursing officer, human resources representative, and hospital attorneys to discuss the approach of building buy-in from the union. You will want to conduct a thorough review of the union agreement to determine whether there is any contract language pertaining to nursing performance and/or peer review.

After conducting the review, you will need to lay out a plan that ensures that all components of the plan have been fleshed out and address any contractual concerns. At that point, you can bring the union to the table.

We recommend that you start with discussions with the union representative to determine what, if any, barriers may exist. Follow these steps to build a foundation of trust, and put yourself in the best position for obtaining buy-in and building trust:

1. Include the union representative in early discussion about peer review.
2. Educate the union representative about the process, standards, and regulatory influence.
3. Provide an opportunity for the union representative to shadow a physician quality leader to better understand how the peer review process works.
4. Provide ongoing communication and updates regarding the plan and the process for implementing peer review.

5. Provide a hospital reference that has incorporated peer review in a union environment. Make sure that the reference hospital and its union rep understand what barriers you are experiencing with the nursing union so that concerns can be addressed.

Your next step is to make an assessment of whether the union supports peer review or is resistant. If you find a supportive attitude, you are on your way to next step, which is to build a plan together (hospital and union) prior to implementation. If the union is resistant, then the time may not be right to incorporate peer review. Work on the union relationship, and try again after you've built a stronger relationship.

Unfortunately, no single, simple solution will guarantee union buy-in, so building the relationship will need to come first.

Reference

The Forces of Magnetism. 2014. Retrieved October 9, 2014, from *www.nursecredentialing.org/Magnet/ProgramOverview/HistoryoftheMagnetProgram/ForcesofMagnetism.*

Aiken, L. 2002. "Superior outcomes for Magnet hospitals: The evidence base." In McClure, M., *Magnet Hospitals Revisited: Attraction and Retention of Professional Nurses.* Washington, DC: American Nurses Publishing.

American Nurses Association. 2004. *Nursing: Scope and Standards of Practice.* Washington, DC: American Nurses Publishing.

Kramer, M., and Schmalenberg, C. 2002. "Staff nurses identify essentials of Magnetism." In McClure, M. *Magnet Hospitals Revisited: Attraction and Retention of Professional Nurses.* Washington, DC: American Nurses Publishing.

McClure, M. L., Poulin, M. A., Sovie, M. D., & Wandelt, M. A. 1983. "Magnet hospitals: Attraction and retention of professional nurses (the original study)" In McClure, M., *Magnet Hospitals Revisited: Attraction and Retention of Professional Nurses.* Washington, DC: American Nurses Publishing.

Chapter 11

Case Studies

Case Study 1 Abdominal Pain

A 68-year-old male patient was admitted with abdominal pain. The patient had a history of congestive heart failure (CHF) and end-stage renal disease. The patient was given an abdominal x-ray, labs, including H+H, and a CT and liver biopsy as part of a diagnostic workup. Four hours postbiopsy, his abdomen was distended, his blood pressure had decreased to 90/60, and his pulse was rapid (110 beats per minute). His hemoglobin decreased from 8 to 5.

The nurse called the physician and reported the increased abdominal pain and vital sign changes but did not recognize the signs and symptoms of postbiopsy intraabdominal bleed. The physician increased pain medication.

Fortunately, when the patient failed to improve, the RN called the rapid response team, who identified the problem and notified the physician, who ordered appropriate interventions, including CT and MRI, which led to an exploratory laparotomy.

Upon receipt of questions from the peer review committee, the RN caring for the patient stated she called the physician to report the critical lab hemoglobin value, but the physician denied receiving that information. There was no documentation in the medical record of the notification.

Refer to Figure 11.1 to see how this case might be scored by the peer review committee.

FIGURE 11.1 | **Scoring of case study 1**

MR # 000001 D/C date 1/22/14 Referral date 1/23/14 Nurse # # 100

Referral source: Check the corresponding box

☑ Screen ❑ Risk ❑ HIM ❑ Nursing ❑ Pharmacy ❑ Pt. Relations ❑ Med Staff ❑ Other ________

Review criteria/Referral issue: Clinical condition changed in patient and not picked up by nursing/delay in calling physician regarding change in patient's condition

Quality screener/Date: 1/26/14 **Date submitted for nurse review:** 1/27/14

Case summary: 68-year-old male admitted with abdominal pain. History of CHF and end-stage renal disease. He had an abdominal x-ray, labs including H+H, and a CT and liver biopsy as part of a diagnostic workup. Four hours post-biopsy his abdomen was distended, his BP had decreased to 90/60, and his pulse was rapid (110 BPM). His hemoglobin decreased from 8 to 5. The nurse called the physician and reported the increased abdominal pain and vital sign changes, but did not recognize the signs/symptoms of post-biopsy intraabdominal bleed. The physician increased pain medication. Fortunately, when the patient failed to improve, the RN called the rapid response team, who identified the problem and notified the physician, who ordered appropriate interventions, including CT and MRI, which led to an exploratory laparotomy.

Key issues for nurse reviewer: 1. Decrease in BP, H&H, and increase in abdominal pain should have been recognized by nurse as a potential post-procedure bleed.
2. Nurse did not document in record or report critical lab value to physician.

To be completed by nurse reviewer

Nurse reviewer: Jane Doe, RN Review date: 1/31/14

Outcome: Check one		
	1	No adverse outcome
✓	2	Minor adverse outcome (complete recovery expected)
	3	Major adverse outcome (complete recovery **NOT** expected)
	4	Catastrophic adverse outcome (e.g., death)

Effect on patient care: Check one		
	1	Care not affected
	2	Increased monitoring/observation (e.g., vital sign checks)
✓	3	Additional treatment/intervention (e.g., IV fluids)
	4	Life sustaining treatment/intervention (e.g., CPR)

FIGURE 11.1 **Scoring of case study 1 (cont'd.)**

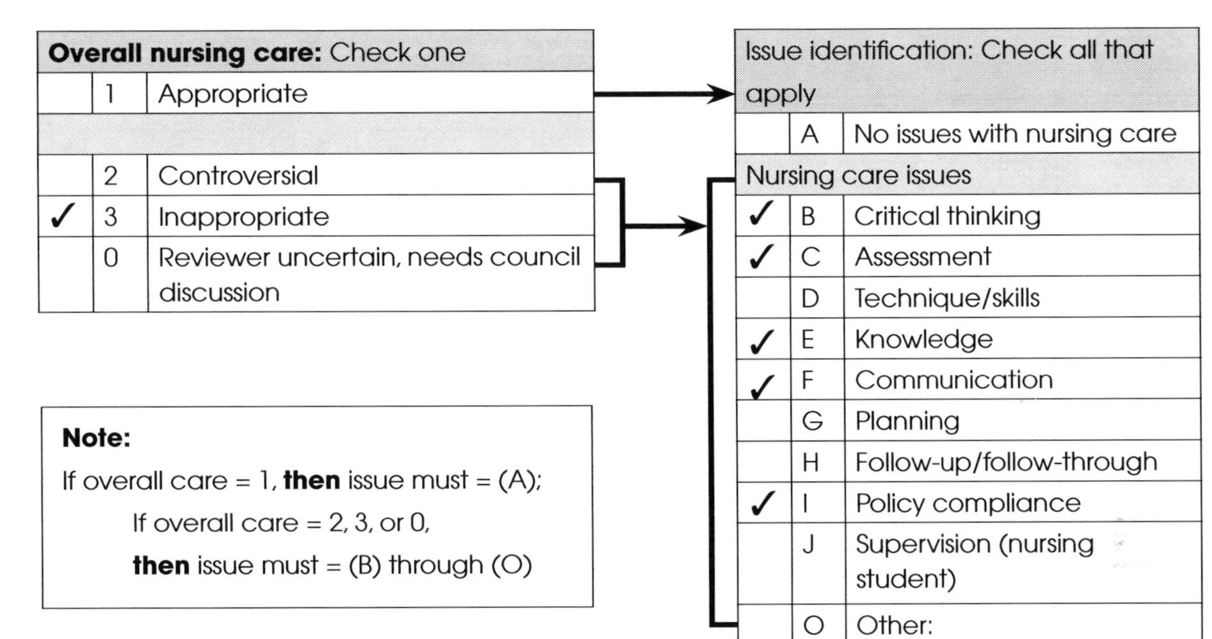

Overall nursing care: Check one		
	1	Appropriate
	2	Controversial
✓	3	Inappropriate
	0	Reviewer uncertain, needs council discussion

Issue identification: Check all that apply		
	A	No issues with nursing care
Nursing care issues		
✓	B	Critical thinking
✓	C	Assessment
	D	Technique/skills
✓	E	Knowledge
✓	F	Communication
	G	Planning
	H	Follow-up/follow-through
✓	I	Policy compliance
	J	Supervision (nursing student)
	O	Other:

Note:
If overall care = 1, **then** issue must = (A);
If overall care = 2, 3, or 0,
then issue must = (B) through (O)

If overall nursing care rated 2, 3, or 0, give a **brief description** of the basis for reviewer findings or concerns:

Nurse did not follow critical lab value policy for reporting and documenting critical labs.

Nurse failed to recognize symptoms of bleed into abdomen.

If overall nursing care rated 2, 3, or 0, **what questions** are to be addressed by the nurse or the council?

After requesting information from the nurse, the RN caring for the patient stated she called the physician to report the critical lab hemoglobin value, but the physician denies receiving that information. There was no documentation in the medical record of the notification.

Nursing documentation: Check all that apply		
	1	No issue with nursing documentation
✓	2	Documentation does not substantiate clinical course and treatment
✓	3	Documentation not timely to communicate with other caregivers
	4	Documentation unreadable
	9	Other:

FIGURE 11.1 | **Scoring of case study 1 (cont'd.)**

Documentation issue description: ______________________________

____

Exemplary nominations: ❑ Nursing care ❑ Nursing documentation

Brief description: ______________________________

Nonnursing care issues: ❑ Potential system or process issue ❑ Potential nursing care issue

Issue description: ______________________________

____

Committee review

Is nurse response needed? ☑ Yes ❑ No

Nurse response: ☑ Discussion with chair ❑ Letter ❑ Committee appearance

Committee final scoring:

Outcome: 2 Documentation: 2/3 Problem identification: B,C,E,F,I

Overall nursing care: 3

	Committee action: Check one	**Date completed**
	No action warranted	
	Nurse self-acknowledged action plan sufficient	
	Educational letter to nurse sufficient	
	Dept. manager discussion of informal improvement plan with nurse	
✓	Dept. manager develops formal improvement plan with monitoring	2/10/14
	Refer to nursing leadership for formal corrective action	

❑ System problem identified—forward to QCC

Date sent ________ Date response ________

Describe system issue ______________________________

❑ Nursing standards issue—forward to nursing leadership

Date sent ________ Date response ________

Describe nursing concern ______________________________

❑ Potential physician issue—forward to medical staff Date sent ________

____

Nursing Peer Review Chair

Case Study 2
Chest Pain

A 75-year-old female was admitted with chest pain for a cardiac catheterization. On admission, her vital signs were stable except for a temperature of 96°C. The patient stated that this temperature was "normal" for her.

In her preprocedure prep, the RN administered sedation (Versed) under physician order, which did not appear to have the desired effect on the patient. After five minutes, the RN contacted the physician, who ordered an additional 2 mg of Versed.

The RN was closely monitoring the patient, who became somnolent and barely responsive and then progressed into respiratory depression. The patient was successfully resuscitated.

In review, it was discovered the department was not accustomed to dealing with hypothermic patients and moderate sedation as were the CRNAs and MDAs who commonly administered sedation. The hospital procedure was modified to reflect the impact of hypothermia, and reeducation was completed.

See Figure 11.2 for an example of how this case might be scored by the peer review committee.

FIGURE 11.2 **Scoring of case study 2**

MR # 000002 D/C date 5/1/14 Referral date 4/28/14 Nurse # 200

Referral source: Check the corresponding box

❑ Screen ❑ Risk ❑ HIM ❑ Nursing ❑ Pharmacy ❑ Pt. Relations ❑ Med Staff

☑ Other Code team

Review criteria/Referral issue: Oversedation leading to respiratory depression

Quality screener/Date: 4/29/14 **Date submitted for nurse review:** 5/2/14

Case summary: On 4/27/14, a 75-year-old female admitted with chest pain for a cardiac catheterization. On admission, her vital signs were stable except for a temperature of 96 degrees. The patient stated that this was "normal" for her. In her preprocedure prep, the RN administered sedation (Versed) under physician order, which didn't seem to have the desired effect. After five minutes, the RN contacted the physician, who ordered an additional 2 mg of Versed. The RN was closely monitoring the patient, who became somnolent and barely responsive, then progressed into respiratory depression. The patient was successfully resuscitated.

Key issues for nurse reviewer: Assessment of patient after sedation administration; hypothermia and the effects on medication absorption; training of staff related to moderate sedation; policy did not specify the effect of hypothermia; supervision of moderate sedation.

To be completed by nurse reviewer

Nurse reviewer: Jane Doe, RN Review date: 5/10/14

Outcome: Check one		
	1	No adverse outcome
✓	2	Minor adverse outcome (complete recovery expected)
	3	Major adverse outcome (complete recovery **NOT** expected)
	4	Catastrophic adverse outcome (e.g., death)

Effect on patient care: Check one		
	1	Care not affected
	2	Increased monitoring/observation (e.g., vital sign checks)
	3	Additional treatment/intervention (e.g., IV fluids)
✓	4	Life sustaining treatment/intervention (e.g., CPR)

FIGURE 11.2 | **Scoring of case study 2 (cont'd.)**

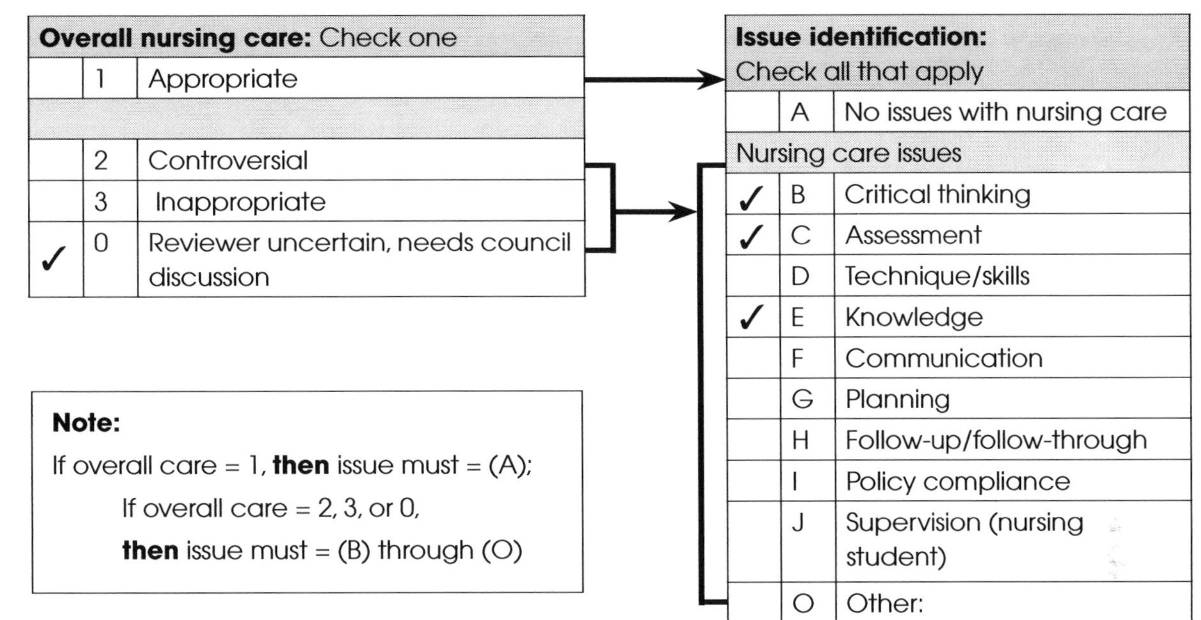

Overall nursing care: Check one		
	1	Appropriate
	2	Controversial
	3	Inappropriate
✓	0	Reviewer uncertain, needs council discussion

Note:
If overall care = 1, **then** issue must = (A);
If overall care = 2, 3, or 0,
then issue must = (B) through (O)

Issue identification: Check all that apply		
	A	No issues with nursing care
Nursing care issues		
✓	B	Critical thinking
✓	C	Assessment
	D	Technique/skills
✓	E	Knowledge
	F	Communication
	G	Planning
	H	Follow-up/follow-through
	I	Policy compliance
	J	Supervision (nursing student)
	O	Other:

If overall nursing care rated 2, 3, or 0, give a brief description of the basis for reviewer findings or concerns:

Nurse performs moderate sedation infrequently and was unfamiliar with the effect of hypothermia during preprocedure sedation.

In review, the nurse performed conscious sedation on a consistent basis, but had not dealt with hypothermic patients.

If overall nursing care rated 2, 3, or 0, what questions are to be addressed by the nurse or the council?

1) Was the overall nursing care appropriate?
2) Revise policy. Is it based on best evidence? Is the hospital policy current and does it mention the affect of hypothermia or any other factors that affect absorption?
3) Who will revise the orientation program and frequency of retraining for moderate sedation?
4) Who needs to be educated and trained on hypothermia?
5) How often should retraining occur for staff, including nurses and physicians, using moderate sedation?

Nursing documentation: Check all that apply		
✓	1	No issue with nursing documentation
	2	Documentation does not substantiate clinical course and treatment
	3	Documentation not timely to communicate with other caregivers
	4	Documentation unreadable
	9	Other:

FIGURE 11.2 **Scoring of case study 2 (cont'd.)**

Documentation issue description: ______________________________

____

Exemplary nominations: ☐ Nursing care ☐ Nursing documentation

Brief description: ______________________________

Nonnursing care issues: ☑ Potential system or process issue ☑ Potential nursing care issue

Issue description: There could be a deficit of knowledge in other areas administering moderate sedation. Are the physicians aware of the effect of hypothermia?

____

Committee review

Is nurse response needed? ☑ Yes ☐ No

Nurse response: ☐ Discussion with chair ☐ Letter ☐ Committee appearance

Committee final scoring:

Outcome: 2 Documentation: 1 Problem identification: E* Overall nursing care: 1

*Patient ID—The nurse demonstrated critical thinking and nursing skills based on current policy. The policy did not reflect hypothermia effect. Nurse was not trained appropriately.

Overall nursing care—Tenured nurse experienced with moderate sedation who did what she should do per current policy, therefore nursing care is deemed appropriate.

Committee action: Check one		**Date completed**
	No action warranted	
✓	Nurse self-acknowledged action plan sufficient	5/12/14
	Educational letter to nurse sufficient	
	Dept. manager discussion of informal improvement plan with nurse	
	Dept. manager develops formal improvement plan with monitoring	
	Refer to nursing leadership for formal corrective action	

FIGURE 11.2 **Scoring of case study 2 (cont'd.)**

☑ System problem identified—forward to QCC

Date sent ____________ Date response 5/12/14

Describe system issue Moderate sedation policy not based on evidence-based practice

❑ Nursing standards issue—forward to nursing leadership

Date sent ____________ Date response ____________

Describe nursing concern ____

☑ Potential physician issue—forward to medical staff Date sent ________

____

Nursing Peer Review Chair

The hospital procedure was modified to reflect the effect of hypothermia and reeducation was completed.

Case Study 3
Patient-Controlled Analgesia (PCA)

A 54-year-old man with a 38-year history of smoking a pack a day is recovering from a bowel resection performed to remove colon cancer. The patient has no additional medical problems and takes no medications. He has been prescribed a morphine PCA pump, with an hourly basal rate of 1 mg morphine, with the ability to administer additional 1-mg doses in divided doses. His oxygen saturation has been running 95% while wearing a 2-liter nasal cannula.

At midnight at the end of the second postoperative day, the patient is found lying on the floor after falling while trying to get up to go to the bathroom. He is not injured, his vital signs are stable, and he is returned to bed.

One hour later, he tells his nurse he has unrelieved, significant pain, after using the maximum allowed dose of PCA morphine. The nurse calls the physician and receives an order to administer a bolus of 2 mg morphine and to increase the PCA to a 2-mg/hour basal hourly rate, with the ability to administer 2 mg additional morphine using the PCA.

At 6 a.m., the patient is found sprawled across the bed, with feet hanging toward the floor. The nurse awakens him enough to reposition him back in the bed. He is groggy, states he has no pain, and falls immediately back to sleep. The nurse is busy so does not check vital signs or the PCA pump. She reports to the next nurse, sharing all the information about the patient's night.

At 8 a.m., the patient cannot be awakened by the day nurse. His respiratory rate is six breaths/minute, heart rate is 52, blood pressure is 74/40, and pulse oximetry saturation is not obtainable. A blood gas is completed, revealing pH 7.22, pCO_2 86, pO_2 60, SaO_2 82% off oxygen. He had removed his cannula and placed it under his pillow.

The PCA protocol states the pump must be checked every two hours, along with vital signs. The patient is given 4 mg of naloxone (Narcan) and awakens in significant pain. His vital signs stabilize and oxygen saturation returns to 98% on a 2-liter nasal cannula. The PCA pump continues at the same dosage. The physician is not notified, since administration of naloxone is part of the PCA protocol.

Refer to Figure 11.3 to see how this case might be scored by the peer review committee.

FIGURE 11.3 **Scoring of case study 3**

MR # 000003 D/C date ____________ Referral date 11/1/14 Nurse # 300

Referral source: Check the corresponding box

❑ Screen ❑ Risk ❑ HIM ☑ Nursing ☑ Pharmacy ❑ Pt. Relations ❑ Med Staff ❑ Other ________

Review criteria/Referral issue: Potential overdose of morphine

Quality screener/Date: 11/3/14 **Date submitted for nurse review:** 11/5/14

Case summary: A 54-year-old man with a 38-year history of smoking a pack a day is recovering from a bowel resection performed to remove colon cancer. He is on a morphine PCA pump, with an hourly basal rate of 1 mg morphine, with the ability to administer additional 1 mg doses in divided doses. His oxygen saturation has been running 95% while wearing a 2-liter nasal cannula.

At midnight at the end of the second post-operative day, the patient is found lying on the floor after falling while trying to get up to go to the bathroom. He is not injured, his vital signs are stable, and he is returned to bed. One hour later, he tells his nurse he has unrelieved, significant pain, after using the maximum allowed dose of PCA morphine. The nurse calls the physician, and receives an order to administer a bolus of 2 mg morphine, and to increase the PCA to a 2 mg/hour basal hourly rate, with the ability to administer 2 mg additional morphine using the PCA.

At 6 a.m., the patient is found sprawled across the bed, with feet hanging toward the floor. The nurse awakens him enough to reposition him back in the bed. He is groggy, states he has no pain, and falls immediately back to sleep.

At 8 a.m., the patient cannot be awakened by the day nurse. His respiratory rate is 6 breaths/minute, heart rate is 52, his blood pressure is 74/40 and his pulse oximetry saturation is not obtainable. A blood gas is completed, revealing pH 7.22, pCO_2 86, pO_2 60, SaO_2 82% off oxygen.

The patient is given 4 mg of naloxone (Narcan) and awakens in significant pain. His vital signs stabilize and oxygen saturation returns to 98% on a 2-liter nasal cannula. The PCA pump continues at the same dosage. The physician is not notified, since administration of naloxone is part of the PCA protocol.

Key issues for nurse reviewer: Did the night nurse provide adequate care?

FIGURE 11.3 **Scoring of case study 3 (cont'd.)**

To be completed by nurse reviewer

Nurse reviewer: Jane Doe, RN   Review date: 11/6/14

Outcome: Check one		
	1	No adverse outcome
✓	2	Minor adverse outcome (complete recovery expected)
	3	Major adverse outcome (complete recovery **NOT** expected)
	4	Catastrophic adverse outcome (e.g., death)

Effect on patient care: Check one		
	1	Care not affected
✓	2	Increased monitoring/ observation (e.g., vital sign checks)
	3	Additional treatment/ intervention (e.g., IV fluids)
	4	Life sustaining treatment/ intervention (e.g., CPR)

Overall nursing care: Check one		
	1	Appropriate
✓	2	Controversial
	3	Inappropriate
	0	Reviewer uncertain, needs council discussion

Note:
If overall care = 1, **then** issue must = (A);
If overall care = 2, 3, or 0, **then** issue must = (B) through (O)

Issue identification: Check all that apply		
	A	No issues with nursing care
Nursing care issues		
	B	Critical thinking
	C	Assessment
	D	Technique/skills
	E	Knowledge
	F	Communication
	G	Planning
	H	Follow-up/follow-through
	I	Policy compliance
	J	Supervision (nursing student)
	O	Other:

If overall nursing care rated 2, 3, or 0, give a **brief description** of the basis for reviewer findings or concerns:
The patient's respiratory status was not closely enough monitored by the night nurse after the medication dose was increased. The patient was already having difficulty tolerating the medication prior to the dosage increase, indicated by his fall on the way to the bathroom.

If overall nursing care rated 2, 3, or 0, **what questions** are to be addressed by the nurse or the council?
N/A—no information needed.

FIGURE 11.3 | **Scoring of case study 3 (cont'd.)**

Nursing documentation: Check all that apply		
	1	No issue with nursing documentation
	2	Documentation does not substantiate clinical course and treatment
	3	Documentation not timely to communicate with other caregivers
	4	Documentation unreadable
✓	9	Other: V/S not recorded, per policy

Documentation issue description: The documentation is complete except for the recording of vital signs per PCA protocol.

Exemplary nominations: ❑ Nursing care ❑ Nursing documentation

Brief description: __________

Nonnursing care issues: ❑ Potential system or process issue ❑ Potential nursing care issue

Issue description: __________

Committee review

Is nurse response needed? ❑ Yes ☑ No

Nurse response: ❑ Discussion with chair ❑ Letter ❑ Committee appearance

Committee final scoring:

Outcome: 2 Documentation: 9 Problem identification: C, H, I Overall nursing care: 3

	Committee action: Check one	**Date completed**
	No action warranted	
	Nurse self-acknowledged action plan sufficient	
	Educational letter to nurse sufficient	
	Dept. manager discussion of informal improvement plan with nurse	
✓	Dept. manager develops formal improvement plan with monitoring	11/15/14
	Refer to nursing leadership for formal corrective action	

FIGURE 11.3 **Scoring of case study 3 (cont'd.)**

❑ System problem identified—forward to QCC

Date sent ____________ Date response ___________

Describe system issue ____

❑ Nursing standards issue—forward to nursing leadership

Date sent ____________ Date response ___________

Describe nursing concern ____

❑ Potential physician issue—forward to medical staff Date sent _______

____

Nursing Peer Review Chair

Case Study 4
Insulin Drip Regulation

An 85-year-old type 2 diabetic woman was transferred to the telemetry unit following a mitral valve replacement two days ago. She has required an insulin drip postoperatively to keep her blood glucose between 80 and 110 mg/dL, in compliance with newly implemented tight glycemic control national standards. She is able to consume two 4-oz containers of apple juice, black coffee, and regular Jell-O prior to transferring to the telemetry unit. All IV fluids, other than insulin drip, were discontinued at 7 a.m. prior to transfer.

The patient's blood glucose is found to be 180 mg/dL prior to breakfast, one hour after consuming the juices and Jell-O. The nurse decides to continue the insulin drip rather than trying to transition the patient to subcutaneous insulin. The insulin drip is increased from 2 units/h to 3 units/h. The patient is given a regular diet for breakfast and eats the entire tray of eggs, bacon, toast, butter, jam, coffee with cream and sugar, orange juice, and grits. One hour later, the patient's point-of-care glucose is 288 mg/dL, so the nurse increases the insulin drip to 4 units/h, per protocol.

The point-of-care blood glucose slowly decreases to 150 mg/dL prior to lunch at noon. The patient consumes a regular diet again at lunch, including spaghetti and meatballs, garlic bread, salad with Italian dressing, green beans with butter, sweet iced tea, and vanilla ice cream. One hour after lunch, the point-of-care glucose is found to be 315 mg/dL, so the insulin drip is increased to 4 units/hour. Continuing with hourly point-of-care readings, the glucose once again drifts down to 145 mg/dL before dinner.

The patient eats another regular diet for dinner, including roast beef with mashed potatoes and gravy, creamed corn, cornbread and butter, fruit cocktail, two cookies, coffee with cream and sugar, and chocolate pudding with whipped cream. One hour following dinner, the point-of-care blood glucose is 298 mg/dL. The insulin drip is increased to 5 units/hour, per protocol. Prior to the bed-time snack at 9 p.m., the point-of-care glucose is 140 mg/dL. The patient is given a ham and cheese sandwich on white bread with mayonnaise and sweet pickles, a bag of potato chips, and a Coke. One hour after the bedtime snack, at 10 p.m., the glucose reading is 300 mg/dL. The insulin drip is increased to 6 units/hour.

At midnight, the point-of-care blood glucose is 200 mg/dL. The patient is given a sleeping pill, as she is bothered by the noise in her unit. At 1 a.m., the patient is not awakened to do a point-of-care reading since she has finally fallen asleep. Just prior to 2 a.m., the staff is startled to hear a lot of noise coming from the patient's room. The patient is having a seizure. Her heart rate has been stable on atenolol. Her point-of-care glucose is found to be 30 mg/dL.

See Figure 11.4 for an example of how this case might be scored by the peer review committee.

FIGURE 11.4 | **Scoring of case study 4**

MR # 000004 D/C date ________ Referral date 6/1/14 Nurse # 400

Referral source: Check the corresponding box

❑ Screen ❑ Risk ❑ HIM ☑ Nursing ☑ Pharmacy ❑ Pt. Relations ❑ Med Staff ❑ Other ______

Review criteria/Referral issue: Nursing care—related to management of insulin.

Quality screener/Date: 6/4/14 **Date submitted for nurse review:** 6/4/14

Case summary: An 85-year-old type II diabetic woman was transferred to the telemetry unit following a mitral valve replacement two days ago. She has required an insulin drip post-operatively to keep her blood glucose between 80–110mg/dL. She is able to consume two 4oz. containers of apple juice, black coffee, and regular Jell-O prior to transferring to the telemetry unit. All IV fluids, other than insulin drip, were discontinued at 7 a.m. prior to transfer.

The patient's blood glucose is found to be 180mg/dL prior to breakfast. The insulin drip is increased from 2 units/hr to 3 units/hr. The patient is given a regular diet for breakfast and eats the entire tray. One hour later, the patient's point-of-care glucose is 288mg/dL, so the nurse increases the insulin drip to 4 units/hr, per protocol.

The point-of-care blood glucose slowly decreases to 150mg/dL prior to lunch at noon. The patient consumes a regular diet again at lunch. One hour after lunch, the point-of-care glucose is found to be 315mg/dL, so the insulin drip is increased to 4 units/hour. Continuing with hourly point-of-care readings, the glucose once again drifts down to 145mg/dL before dinner.

FIGURE 11.4 | **Scoring of case study 4 (cont'd.)**

Case summary (cont.):

The patient eats another regular diet for dinner. One hour following dinner, the point of care blood glucose is 298mg/dL. The insulin drip is increased to 5 units/hr, per protocol. Prior to the bedtime snack at 9 p.m., the point-of-care glucose is 140mg/dL. One hour after the bedtime snack, at 10 p.m., the glucose reading is 300mg/dL. The insulin drip is increased to 6 units/hr.

At midnight, the point-of-care blood glucose is 200mg/dL. The patient is given a sleeping pill, as she is bothered by the noise in her unit. At 1 a.m., the patient is not awakened to do a point-of-care reading since she has finally fallen asleep. Just prior to 2 a.m., the staff is startled to hear a lot of noise coming from the patient's room. The patient is having a seizure. Her heart rate has been stable on atenolol. Her point-of-care glucose is found to be 30mg/dL.

Key issues for nurse reviewer: Did the day nurse provide adequate care? Did the night nurse provide adequate care? (To be reviewed on separate form.)

To be completed by nurse reviewer

Nurse reviewer: Jane Doe, RN

Review date: 6/10/14

Outcome: Check one		
	1	No adverse outcome
✓	2	Minor adverse outcome (complete recovery expected)
	3	Major adverse outcome (complete recovery **NOT** expected)
	4	Catastrophic adverse outcome (e.g., death)

Effect on patient care: Check one		
	1	Care not affected
	2	Increased monitoring/ observation (e.g., vital sign checks)
	3	Additional treatment/ intervention (e.g., IV fluids)
✓	4	Life sustaining treatment/ intervention (e.g., CPR)

FIGURE 11.4 **Scoring of case study 4 (cont'd.)**

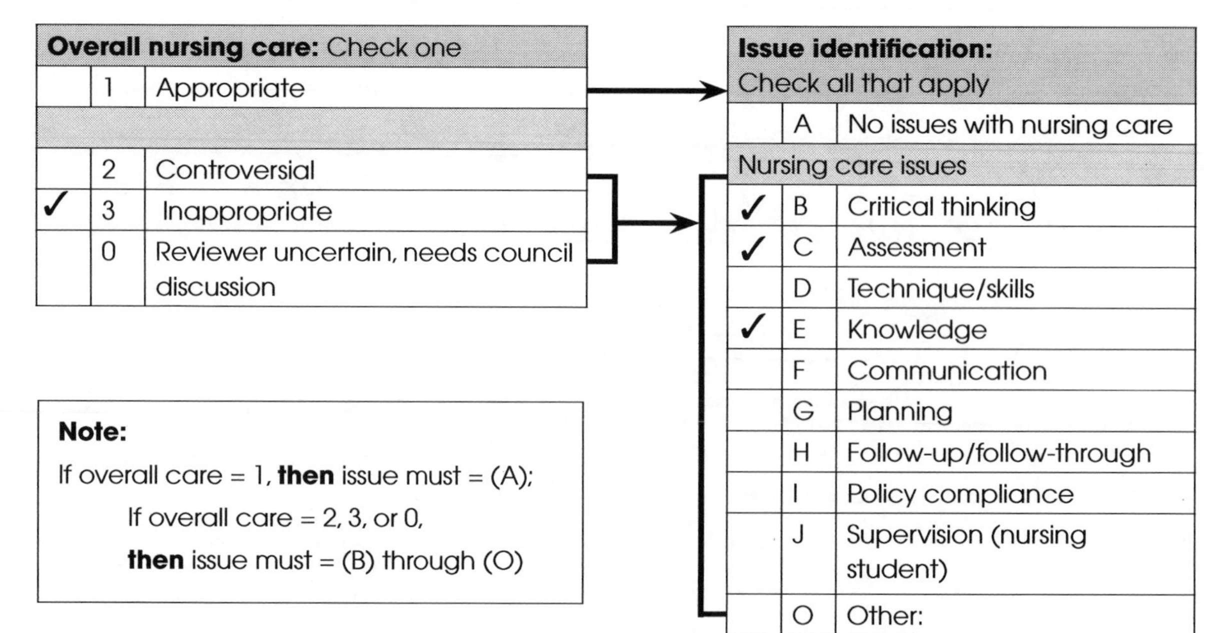

Overall nursing care: Check one		
	1	Appropriate
	2	Controversial
✓	3	Inappropriate
	0	Reviewer uncertain, needs council discussion

Issue identification: Check all that apply		
	A	No issues with nursing care
Nursing care issues		
✓	B	Critical thinking
✓	C	Assessment
	D	Technique/skills
✓	E	Knowledge
	F	Communication
	G	Planning
	H	Follow-up/follow-through
	I	Policy compliance
	J	Supervision (nursing student)
	O	Other:

Note:
If overall care = 1, **then** issue must = (A);
If overall care = 2, 3, or 0,
then issue must = (B) through (O)

If overall nursing care rated 2, 3, or 0, give a **brief description** of the basis for reviewer findings or concerns:

The day nurse should have approached the physician for subcutaneous insulin orders for a long-acting basal insulin (glargine, detemir, or NPH), scheduled mealtime coverage using short-acting insulin if glargine or detemir were used, and supplemental short-acting insulin for any elevations in blood glucose found to be present prior to meals. The patient should also have been given a controlled carbohydrate diet, rather than a regular diet. By providing a regular diet, the patient received too many carbohydrates and the insulin drip had to be used to manage the rise in blood glucose following meals. This is a potentially dangerous practice, as when meals cease, the carbohydrate load stops and the need for insulin is markedly reduced.

Patients who are eating meals are best managed using subcutaneous insulin, which can more accurately be used to mimic the body's normal pattern of insulin secretion. Controlled carbohydrate diet helps to stabilize blood glucose as well.

If overall nursing care rated 2, 3, or 0, **what questions** are to be addressed by the nurse or the council?

N/A—no questions.

FIGURE 11.4 | **Scoring of case study 4 (cont'd.)**

Nursing documentation: Check all that apply		
✓	1	No issue with nursing documentation
	2	Documentation does not substantiate clinical course and treatment
	3	Documentation not timely to communicate with other caregivers
	4	Documentation unreadable
	9	Other:

Documentation issue description: No issues noted with documentation.

Exemplary nominations: ❑ Nursing care ❑ Nursing documentation

Brief description: ______

Nonnursing care issues: ❑ Potential system or process issue ❑ Potential nursing care issue

Issue description: ______

Committee review

Is nurse response needed? ❑ Yes ☑ No

Nurse response: ❑ Discussion with chair ❑ Letter ❑ Committee appearance

Committee final scoring:

Outcome: 2 Documentation: 1 Problem identification: B, C, E Overall nursing care: 3

Committee action: Check one		**Date completed**
	No action warranted	
	Nurse self-acknowledged action plan sufficient	
	Educational letter to nurse sufficient	
	Dept. manager discussion of informal improvement plan with nurse	
✓	Dept. manager develops formal improvement plan with monitoring	6/20/14
	Refer to nursing leadership for formal corrective action	

FIGURE 11.4 **Scoring of case study 4 (cont'd.)**

❑ System problem identified—forward to QCC

Date sent ____________ Date response ___________

Describe system issue ____

❑ Nursing standards issue—forward to nursing leadership

Date sent ____________ Date response ___________

Describe nursing concern ____

❑ Potential physician issue—forward to medical staff Date sent ________

____

Nursing Peer Review Chair